McGraw-Hill Education

MCAT

2 FULL-LENGTH PRACTICE TESTS

2015

McGraw-Hill Education
MCAT
Test Preparation Series

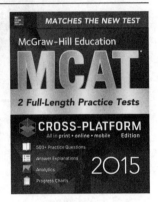

- Biomolecules
- Molecules, Cells, and Organs
- Systems of Tissues and Organs

- Physical Foundations of Biological Systems
- Chemical Foundations of Biological Systems

- Perception and Response
- Behavior
- Self and Others
- Social Structure
- Social Strata
- Critical Analysis and Reasoning Skills

- Practice Test 1
- Answers and Explanations
- Practice Test 2
- Answers and Explanations

McGraw-Hill Education

MCAT

2 FULL-LENGTH PRACTICE TESTS

2015

George J. Hademenos, PhD

Candice McCloskey Campbell, PhD

Shaun Murphree, PhD

Amy B. Wachholtz, PhD

Jennifer M. Warner, PhD

Kathy A. Zahler, MS

Thomas A. Evangelist, MA   Contributor

New York   Chicago   San Francisco   Athens   London   Madrid
Mexico City   Milan   New Delhi   Singapore   Sydney   Toronto

2 3 4 5 6 7 8 9 10 RHR/RHR 1 0 9 8 7 6 5

ISBN   978-0-07-182441-5
MHID   0-07-182441-3

e-ISBN   978-0-07-182569-6
e-MHID   0-07-182569-X

Library of Congress Control Number 2014936768

MCAT is a registered trademark of the Association of American Medical Colleges, which was not involved in the production of, and does not endorse, this product.

Amy B. Wachholtz, PhD, would like to thank Christopher Ayala, MA, for assistance with fact checking and editing the behavioral and social sciences material in this volume.

McGraw-Hill Education products are available at special quantity discounts to use as premiums and sales promotions or for use in corporate training programs. To contact a representative, please visit the Contact Us pages at www.mhprofessional.com.

This book is printed on acid-free paper.

Contents

MCAT PRACTICE TEST 1

MCAT PRACTICE TEST 2

About the Authors

George J. Hademenos, PhD, is a former Visiting Assistant Professor of Physics at the University of Dallas. He received his BS from Angelo State University, received his MS and PhD from the University of Texas at Dallas, and completed postdoctoral fellowships in nuclear medicine at the University of Massachusetts Medical Center and in radiological sciences/biomedical physics at UCLA Medical Center. His research interests have involved potential applications of physics to the biological and medical sciences, particularly with cerebrovascular diseases and stroke. He has published his work in journals such as *American Scientist, Physics Today, Neurosurgery,* and *Stroke.* In addition, he has written several books including *The Physics of Cerebrovascular Diseases*: *Biophysical Mechanisms of Development, Diagnosis and Therapy,* and *Schaum's Outline of Biology.* He currently teaches general and advanced physics courses.

Candice McCloskey Campbell, PhD, received her doctorate in organic chemistry from Georgia Tech in 1985. She has been teaching at the undergraduate level since 1987. She currently teaches at Georgia Perimeter College in Dunwoody, Georgia. Her professional work has been in synthetic organic chemistry and mechanistic organic chemistry. She has been active with the Two-Year College Chemistry Consortium to enhance the chemistry curriculum at the two-year college level.

Shaun Murphree, PhD, is Professor and Chair of Chemistry at Allegheny College in Meadville, Pennsylvania. He received a BA in chemistry from Colgate University (Hamilton, New York) and a PhD in organic chemistry from Emory University (Atlanta, Georgia), and he conducted post-doctoral study at Wesleyan University (Middletown, Connecticut). His current research interests include microwave-assisted organic synthesis (MAOS), synthetic methodology, and heterocyclic synthesis. In addition to the present work, he has coauthored a monograph on microwave chemistry, several chapters and reviews on heterocyclic synthesis, and numerous articles in both the synthetic chemistry and chemistry education literature.

Amy B. Wachholtz, PhD, MDiv, MS, is an Assistant Professor of Psychiatry at the University of Massachusetts Medical School and the Director of Health Psychology at UMass Memorial Medical Center. Dr. Wachholtz graduated with a Master of Divinity degree from Boston University, where she specialized in bioethics. She then continued her education to earn a Master's and PhD in clinical psychology from Bowling Green State University, where she had a dual specialization in behavioral medicine and psychology of religion. She completed internship through fellowship at Duke University Medical Center, where she focused on medical psychology. She has also completed a post-doctoral MS degree in psychopharmacology. Dr. Wachholtz has multiple funded research projects with her primary focus on (1) bio-psycho-social-spiritual model of chronic pain disorders and (2) the complexities of treating of comorbid pain and opioid addiction in both acute pain and chronic pain situations. She enjoys teaching students from a variety of health disciplines, both in the classroom and on the clinical floors of UMass Memorial Medical Center Hospitals.

Jennifer M. Warner, PhD, is the Director of the University Honors Program and a member of the faculty in the Department of Biological Sciences at the University of North Carolina at Charlotte. She received her BS in Biology from the University of North Carolina at Chapel Hill, her MS in Biology with a focus in microbiology from the University of North Carolina at Charlotte, and her PhD in Curriculum and Teaching from the University of North Carolina at Greensboro. Her current research interests revolve around variables that influence student success and retention in the sciences. She currently teaches a variety of courses including principles of biology, human biology, the nature of science, and pathogenic bacteriology.

Kathy A. Zahler, MS, is a widely published author and textbook writer. She has authored or coauthored numerous McGraw-Hill Education preparation guides for tests, including the GRE®, the Miller Analogies Test, the Test of Essential Academic Skills (TEAS®), and the Test Assessing Secondary Completion™ (TASC™).

How to Use the McGraw-Hill Education MCAT Preparation Series

Welcome to the McGraw-Hill Education MCAT Preparation series. You've made the decision to pursue a medical career, you've studied hard, you've taken and passed the most difficult science courses, and now you must succeed on this very tough exam. We're here to help you.

This series has been created by a dedicated team of scientists, teachers, and test-prep experts. Together, they have helped thousands of students to score high on all kinds of exams, from rigorous science tests to difficult essay-writing assignments. They have pooled their knowledge, experience, and test-taking expertise to make this the most effective self-study MCAT preparation program available.

The four books in this series contain a wealth of features to help you do your best. The four volumes are organized as follows:

MCAT Biological and Biochemical Foundations of Living Systems provides:

➤ **A general introduction to the MCAT,** including basic facts about the structure and format of the test and the kinds of questions you will encounter.

➤ **Important test-taking strategies** that can help you raise your score.

➤ **An in-depth review of all the topics tested in Part 1 of the exam: Biological and Biochemical Foundations of Living Systems.** This is the exam section that assesses your knowledge of foundational concepts in biology and biochemistry, and your understanding of how biological processes function both separately and together in living systems, including the human body.

➤ **Minitests modeled on Part 1 of the exam.** These practice exams are designed to simulate the actual MCAT in format and degree of difficulty. The questions ask you to use your scientific research and reasoning skills to solve problems demonstrating your mastery of the skills required for success in medical school.

MCAT Chemical and Physical Foundations of Biological Systems provides:

➤ **A general introduction to the MCAT,** including basic facts about the structure and format of the test and the kinds of questions you will encounter.

➤ **Important test-taking strategies** that can help you raise your score.

➤ **An in-depth review of all the topics tested in Part 2 of the exam: Chemical and Physical Foundations of Biological Systems.** This is the exam section that assesses your knowledge of foundational concepts in organic chemistry and physics, and your understanding of how chemical and physical processes function both separately and together in living systems, including the human body.

➤ **Minitests modeled on Part 2 of the exam.** These practice exams are designed to simulate the actual MCAT in format and degree of difficulty. The questions ask you to use your scientific research and reasoning skills to solve problems demonstrating your mastery of the skills required for success in medical school.

MCAT Behavioral and Social Sciences & Critical Analysis provides:

➤ **A general introduction to the MCAT,** including basic facts about the structure and format of the test and the kinds of questions you will encounter.

➤ **An in-depth review of all the topics tested in Parts 3 and 4 of the exam: Psychological, Social, and Biological Foundations of Behavior and Critical Analysis and Reasoning Skills.** Part 3 of the exam tests your knowledge of basic concepts in psychology and sociology that are important for understanding how behavioral and sociocultural factors affect health outcomes and the provision of health care. Part 4 of the exam tests your ability to analyze, evaluate, and apply information from reading passages in a wide range of social sciences and humanities areas.

➤ **Minitests modeled on Parts 3 and 4 of the exam.** These practice exams are designed to simulate the actual MCAT in format and degree of difficulty. The questions ask you to use your scientific research and reasoning skills to solve problems that demonstrate your mastery of the skills required for success in medical school.

MCAT 2 Full-Length Practice Tests provides:

➤ **A general introduction to the MCAT,** including basic facts about the structure and format of the test and the kinds of questions you will encounter.

➤ **Important test-taking strategies** that can help you raise your score.

➤ **Two full-length practice MCAT tests** designed to simulate the real exam in structure, format, and degree of difficulty. Of course, these practice tests can provide only an approximation of how well you will do on the actual MCAT. However, if you approach them as you would the real test, they should give you a very good idea of how well you are prepared.

➤ **Explanations for every question.** After you take each test, read carefully through these explanations, paying special attention to those you answered incorrectly or had to guess on. If necessary, go back and reread the corresponding subject review sections in the earlier volumes.

Different people have different ways of preparing for a test like the MCAT. You must find a preparation method that suits your schedule and your learning style. We have tried to make this series flexible enough for you to use in a way that works best for you, but to succeed on this extremely rigorous exam, there is no substitute for serious, intensive review and study. The more time and effort you devote to preparing, the better your chances of achieving your MCAT goals.

Introducing the MCAT

MCAT BASICS

The Medical College Admission Test (MCAT) is a standardized exam that is used to assess applicants to medical schools. The test is sponsored by the Association of American Medical Colleges (AAMC) in cooperation with its member schools. It is required as part of the admissions process by most US medical schools. The test is administered by Prometric, a private firm that is a leading provider of technology-based testing and assessment services.

The questions on the MCAT are basically designed to measure your problem-solving and critical-thinking skills. Two test sections assess your mastery of fundamental concepts in biology, biochemistry, general chemistry, organic chemistry, and physics. A third section tests your understanding of concepts in psychology, sociology, and biology that are important to understanding how behavioral and sociocultural factors affect health outcomes and the provision of healthcare. For most questions in these sections, choosing the correct answer requires more than just a rote response; you must calculate a solution, interpret and evaluate given data, or apply a particular scientific principle to a given situation. You will need to demonstrate that you can reason scientifically and employ the principles of research methodology and statistics. There is also a fourth section that tests your ability to analyze, evaluate, and apply information from reading passages on topics in ethics, philosophy, cross-cultural studies, and population health.

According to the AAMC, the skills tested on the MCAT are those identified by medical professionals and educators as essential for success in medical school and in a career as a physician. The importance of the biological, biochemical, and physical sciences is self-evident. Psychological and sociological concepts are included, according to the AAMC, because "knowledge of the behavioral and social determinants of health and wellness [is] becoming more important in medical education," and "tomorrow's doctors need to know [these concepts] in order to serve a more diverse population and to understand the impact of behavior on health and wellness."

THE COMPUTERIZED TEST FORMAT

You will take the MCAT on a computer. You will view the questions on the computer screen and indicate your answers by clicking on on-screen answer ovals. As you work through the on-screen questions, you will be able to highlight relevant portions of the reading passages for easy reference. You will also be able to strike out answer choices that you know are incorrect. This will help you use the process of elimination to pick the correct answer. You will also be allowed to make notes on scratch paper (although all of your notes will be collected at the end of the test). Within each test section, you will be able to go back, review questions that you have already answered, and change your answer if you decide to do so. However, once you have finished a test section, you cannot go back to it and make any changes.

Don't be concerned if you are not a whiz with computers; the skills required are minimal, and in any case, on test day you will have the opportunity to access a computer tutorial that will show you exactly what you need to do.

WHERE AND WHEN TO TAKE THE MCAT

The MCAT is offered at approximately 275 sites in the United States (including the US territories of Puerto Rico and the Virgin Islands) and at 12 sites in Canada. All of these sites are testing labs operated by Prometric. The test is also offered at numerous locations outside North America, including sites in Europe, Great Britain, the Middle East, Africa, Asia, and Australia.

There are 22 test dates every year. Two of the dates are in January, and the rest are in the period from April through early September. Most test dates are weekdays, but a few are Saturdays. On some dates, the test is given only in the morning; on others, it is given only in the afternoon. On a few dates, the test is given in both morning and afternoon sessions.

It is a good idea to take the MCAT in the spring or summer of the year before the fall in which you plan to enroll in medical school. That way, you have enough time to submit your scores to meet the schools' application deadlines.

For up-to-date lists of testing sites and also for upcoming test dates, make sure to check the official MCAT website at www.aamc.org/mcat.

HOW TO REGISTER FOR THE MCAT

You can register for the MCAT online at www.aamc.org/mcat. Online registration for each test date begins six months prior to that date. Registration is available until two weeks before the test date. It's a good idea to register early, because seating at the testing centers may be limited and you want to make sure you get a seat at the center of your choice. When you register, you are charged a fee, which you can pay by credit card. If you wish to change your test date, you can do so online.

TAKING THE MCAT MORE THAN ONCE

If your MCAT score is lower than expected, you may want to take the test again. You can take the MCAT up to three times in the same year. However, the AAMC recommends retesting only if you have a good reason to think that you will do better the next time. For example, you might do better if, when you first took the test, you were ill, or you made mistakes in keying in your answers, or your academic background in one or more of the test subjects was inadequate.

If you are considering retesting, you should also find out how your chosen medical schools evaluate multiple scores. Some schools give equal weight to all MCAT scores; others average scores together, and still others look only at the highest scores. Check with admissions officers before making a decision.

YOUR MCAT SCORES

When you take the MCAT, your work on each of the four test sections first receives a "raw score." The raw score is calculated based on the number of questions you answer correctly. No points are deducted for questions answered incorrectly. Each raw score is then converted into a scaled score. Using scaled scores helps make test-takers' scores comparable from one version of the MCAT to another. For each of the four sections, scaled scores range from 1 (lowest) to 15 (highest).

Your score report will be mailed to you approximately 30 days after you take the MCAT. You will also be able to view your scores on the online MCAT Testing History (THx) System as soon as they become available. (For details on the THx system, see the MCAT website.) MCAT score reports also include percentile rankings that show how well you did in comparison to others who took the same test.

HOW MEDICAL SCHOOLS USE MCAT SCORES

Medical college admission committees emphasize that MCAT scores are only one of several criteria that they consider when evaluating applicants. When making their decisions, they also consider students' college and university grades, recommendations, interviews, and involvement and participation in extracurricular or health care–related activities that, in the opinion of the admission committee, illustrate maturity, motivation, dedication, and other positive personality traits that are of value to a physician. If the committee is unfamiliar with the college you attend, they may pay more attention than usual to your MCAT scores.

There is no hard-and-fast rule about what schools consider to be an acceptable MCAT score. A few schools accept a score as low as 4, but many require scores of 10 or higher. To get into a top-ranked school, you generally need scores of 12 or higher. A high score on the Writing Sample may compensate for any weaknesses in communication skills noted on the application or at an interview.

Note that many medical schools do not accept MCAT scores that are more than three years old.

REPORTING SCORES TO MEDICAL SCHOOLS

Your MCAT scores are automatically reported to the American Medical College Application Service (AMCAS), the nonprofit application processing service used by nearly all U.S. medical schools. When you use this service, you complete and submit a single application, rather than separate applications to each of your chosen schools. Your scores are submitted to your designated schools along with your application. There is a fee for using AMCAS. If you wish to submit your scores to other application services or to programs that do not participate in AMCAS, you can do so through the online MCAT Testing History (THx) System.

FOR FURTHER INFORMATION

For further information about the MCAT, visit the official MCAT website at

www.aamc.org/mcat

For questions about registering for the test, reporting and interpreting scores, and similar issues, you may also contact:

Association of American Medical Colleges
Medical College Admission Test
655 K Street, NW, Suite 100
Washington, DC 20001-2399

THE FORMAT OF THE TEST

The MCAT consists of four separately timed sections as outlined in the following chart.

MCAT: Format of the Test		
Section	Number of Questions	Time Allowed (minutes)
1. Biological and Biochemical Foundations of Living Systems *Break: 10 minutes*	65	95
2. Chemical and Physical Foundations of Biological Systems *Break: 10 minutes*	65	95
3. Psychological, Social, and Biological Foundations of Behavior *Break: 10 minutes*	65	95
4. Critical Analysis and Reasoning Skills	60	90
Totals	255	375 (= 6 hours, 15 minutes)

WHAT IS TESTED IN THE SCIENCE SECTIONS

The natural sciences sections of the MCAT (Sections 1 and 2) test your mastery of the concepts and principles of biology, biochemistry, general chemistry, organic chemistry, and physics as they apply to living systems, including the human body.

The behavioral and social sciences section of the MCAT (Section 3) tests your understanding of the behavioral and sociocultural factors that play a role in health care. These three sections have three main organizing principles:

1. **Foundational concepts:** what the AAMC calls the "big ideas" in the sciences that underlie the subjects taught in medical school
2. **Content categories:** the topics that support the foundational concepts
3. **Scientific inquiry and reasoning skills:** the skills needed to solve scientific problems

Foundational Concepts and Content Categories

According to the AAMS, the foundational concepts and categories for sections 1, 2, and 3 of the MCAT are as follows:

BIOLOGICAL AND BIOCHEMICAL FOUNDATIONS OF LIVING SYSTEMS

Foundational Concept 1: *Biomolecules have unique properties that determine how they contribute to the structure and function of cells and how they participate in the processes necessary to maintain life.*

Content categories:

➤ Structure and function of proteins and their constituent amino acids

➤ Transmission of genetic information from the gene to the protein

➤ Transmission of heritable information from generation to generation and the processes that increase genetic diversity

➤ Principles of bioenergetics and fuel molecule metabolism

Foundational Concept 2: *Highly organized assemblies of molecules, cells, and organs interact to carry out the functions of living organisms.*

Content categories:

➤ Assemblies of molecules, cells, and groups of cells within single cellular and multicellular organisms

➤ Structure, growth, physiology, and genetics of prokaryotes and viruses

➤ Processes of cell division, differentiation, and specialization

Foundational Concept 3: *Complex systems of tissues and organs sense the internal and external environments of multicellular organisms and, through integrated functioning, maintain a stable internal environment within an ever-changing external environment.*

Content categories:

➤ Structure and functions of the nervous and endocrine systems and ways in which these systems coordinate the organ systems

➤ Structure and integrative functions of the main organ systems

CHEMICAL AND PHYSICAL FOUNDATIONS OF BIOLOGICAL SYSTEMS

Foundational Concept 4: *Complex living organisms transport materials, sense their environment, process signals, and respond to changes using processes that can be understood in terms of physical principles.*

Content categories:

➤ Translational motion, forces, work, energy, and equilibrium in living systems

➤ Importance of fluids for the circulation of blood, gas movement, and gas exchange

➤ Electrochemistry and electrical circuits and their elements

➤ How light and sound interact with matter

➤ Atoms, nuclear decay, electronic structure, and atomic chemical behavior

Foundational Concept 5: *The principles that govern chemical interactions and reactions form the basis for a broader understanding of the molecular dynamics of living systems.*

Content categories:

➤ Unique nature of water and its solutions

➤ Nature of molecules and intermolecular interactions

➤ Separation and purification methods

➤ Structure, function, and reactivity of biologically relevant molecules

➤ Principles of chemical thermodynamics and kinetics

PSYCHOLOGICAL, SOCIAL, AND BIOLOGICAL FOUNDATIONS OF BEHAVIOR

Foundational Concept 6: *Biological, psychological, and sociocultural factors influence the ways that individuals perceive, think about, and react to the world.*

Content categories:

➤ Sensing the environment

➤ Making sense of the environment

➤ Responding to the world

Foundational Concept 7: *Biological, psychological, and sociocultural factors influence behavior and behavior change.*

Content categories:

➤ Individual influences on behavior

➤ Social processes that influence human behavior

➤ Attitude and behavior change

Foundational Concept 8: *Psychological, sociocultural, and biological factors influence the way we think about ourselves and others, as well as how we interact with others.*

Content categories:

➤ Self-identity

➤ Social thinking

➤ Social interactions

Foundational Concept 9: *Cultural and social differences influence well-being.*

Content categories:

➤ Understanding social structure

➤ Demographic characteristics and processes

Foundational Concept 10: *Social stratification and access to resources influence well-being.*

Content category:

➤ Social inequality

Scientific Inquiry and Reasoning Skills

The scientific inquiry and reasoning skills that are tested on Sections 1, 2, and 3 of the MCAT are as follows:

➤ **Skill 1:** Knowledge of Scientific Concepts and Principles

➤ **Skill 2:** Scientific Reasoning and Evidence-Based Problem Solving

➤ **Skill 3:** Reasoning About the Design and Execution of Research

➤ **Skill 4:** Data-Based and Statistical Reasoning

To demonstrate mastery of **Skill 1: Knowledge of Scientific Concepts and Principles,** you need to be able to recall and apply basic scientific concepts and principles to solve problems in science. In many cases, you will need to analyze and interpret information presented in diagrams, charts, graphs, and formulas.

To demonstrate mastery of **Skill 2: Scientific Reasoning and Evidence-Based Problem Solving,** you need to be able to understand and use scientific theories, to propose hypotheses, and to analyze scientific models or research studies in order to identify assumptions, make predictions, and draw conclusions.

To demonstrate mastery of **Skill 3: Reasoning About the Design and Execution of Research,** you need to be able to identify appropriate research designs for investigating specified research questions, to critique and evaluate those designs, to predict results, and to recognize ethical issues involved in research.

To demonstrate mastery of **Skill 4: Data-Based and Statistical Reasoning,** you need to be able to interpret data or to describe or evaluate the results of a research study using statistical concepts.

WHAT IS TESTED IN CRITICAL ANALYSIS AND REASONING SKILLS

The Critical Analysis and Reasoning Skills section of the MCAT (Section 4) tests your ability to comprehend information in a reading passage, to analyze and evaluate arguments and supporting evidence, and to apply concepts and ideas to new situations. The passages in this section cover a wide range of topics in both the social sciences and the humanities. You may encounter readings in philosophy, ethics, cultural studies, and similar topics. All the information you need to answer questions will be provided in the passage; no outside knowledge of the topics is required.

According to the AAMC, the questions in the Critical Analysis and Reasoning Skills section test the following four specific skills:

➤ **Comprehension:** the ability to understand new information or to view facts or ideas in a new light.

➤ **Evaluation:** the ability to analyze ideas or arguments presented in a passage and to make judgments about their reasonableness, their credibility, and the soundness of supporting evidence.

➤ **Application:** the ability to apply information in a passage to new conditions or situations and to predict possible outcomes.

➤ **Incorporation of Information:** the ability to consider how new information affects the ideas presented in a passage, for example, whether it strengthens or weakens an argument or a hypothesis.

GENERAL TEST-TAKING STRATEGIES

The following sections present some general test-taking strategies that apply to the multiple-choice questions on the MCAT. These strategies can help you to gain valuable points when you take the actual test.

Take Advantage of the Multiple-Choice Format

All of the questions on the MCAT are in the multiple-choice format, which you have undoubtedly seen many times before. That means that for every question, the correct answer is right in front of you. All you have to do is pick it out from among three incorrect choices, called "distracters." Consequently, you can use the process of elimination to rule out incorrect answer choices. The more answers you rule out, the easier it is to make the right choice.

Answer Every Question

Recall that on the MCAT, there is no penalty for choosing a wrong answer. Therefore, if you do not know the answer to a question, you have nothing to lose by guessing. So make sure that you answer every question. If time is running out and you still have not answered some questions, make sure to enter an answer for the questions that you have not attempted. With luck, you may be able to pick up a few extra points, even if your guesses are totally random.

Make Educated Guesses

What differentiates great test takers from merely good ones is the ability to guess in such a way as to maximize the chance of guessing correctly. The way to do this is to use the process of elimination. Before you guess, try to eliminate one or more of the answer choices. That way, you can make an educated guess, and you have a better chance of picking the correct answer. Odds of one out of two or one out of three are better than one out of four!

Go with Your Gut

In those cases where you're not 100% sure of the answer you are choosing, it is often best to go with your gut feeling and stick with your first answer. If you decide to change that answer and pick another one, you may well pick the wrong answer because you have over-thought the problem. More often than not, if you know something about the subject, your first answer is likely to be the correct one.

Take Advantage of Helpful Computer Functions

On the MCAT, you have access to certain computer functions that can make your work easier. As you work through the on-screen questions, you are able to highlight relevant portions of the reading passages. This helps you save time when you need to find facts or details to support your answer choices. You are also able to cross out answer choices that you know are incorrect. This helps you use the process of elimination to pick the correct answer.

Use the Scratch Paper Provided

The MCAT is an all-computerized test, so there is no test booklet for you to write in. However, you are given scratch paper, so use it to your advantage. Jot down notes, make calculations, and write out an outline for each of your essays. Be aware, however, that you cannot remove the scratch paper from the test site. All papers are collected from you before you leave the room.

Because you cannot write on the actual MCAT, don't get into the habit of writing notes to yourself on the test pages of this book. Use separate scratch paper instead. Consider it an opportunity to learn to use scratch paper effectively.

Keep Track of the Time

Make sure that you're on track to answer all of the questions within the time allowed. With so many questions to answer in a short time period, you're not going to have a lot of time to spare. Keep an eye on your watch or on the computerized timer provided.

Do not spend too much time on any one question. If you find yourself stuck for more than a minute or two on a question, then you should make your best guess and move on. If you have time left over at the end of the section, you can return to the question and review your answer. However, if time runs out, don't give the question another thought. You need to save your focus for the rest of the test.

Don't Panic if Time Runs Out

If you pace yourself and keep track of your progress, you should not run out of time. If you do, however, run out of time, don't panic. Because there is no guessing penalty and you have nothing to lose by doing so, enter answers to all the remaining questions. If you are able to make educated guesses, you will probably be able to improve your score. However, even random guesses may help you pick up a few points. In order to know how to handle this situation if it happens to you on the test, make sure you observe the time limits when you take the practice tests. Guessing well is a skill that comes with practice, so incorporate it into your preparation program.

If Time Permits, Review Questions You Were Unsure Of

Within each test section, the computer allows you to return to questions you have already answered and change your answer if you decide to do so. (However, once you have completed an entire section, you cannot go back to it and make changes.) If time permits, you may want to take advantage of this function to review questions you were unsure of or to check for careless mistakes.

About the Practice Tests

The Practice Tests in this volume are designed to help you determine your readiness to take the actual MCAT. Each test has four separately timed sections as shown in the chart.

Section	Number of Questions	Time Allowed (minutes)
1. Biological and Biochemical Foundations of Living Systems	65	95
Break: 10 minutes		
2. Chemical and Physical Foundations of Biological Systems	65	95
Break: 10 minutes		
3. Psychological, Social, and Biological Foundations of Behavior	65	95
Break: 10 minutes		
4. Critical Analysis and Reasoning Skills	60	90
Totals	255	375 (= 6 hours, 15 minutes)

The questions are designed to match the real exam as closely as possible in format and degree of difficulty. If you approach these tests as you would the real exam, your results will give you a good idea of how well you would score if you took the real MCAT today.

Each test is followed by complete explanations for every question. Study the explanations carefully, particularly for questions that you missed or that you found difficult.

Following each set of explanations is an Evaluation Chart. Use it to measure your test-taking readiness and to pinpoint content areas that you may need to review again before taking the real exam.

How to Use the Practice Tests

The following pages present two full-length practice MCATs. The questions have been designed to match real MCAT questions as closely as possible in terms of format and degree of difficulty. If you are at the beginning of your MCAT preparation, you can use these tests as launching-points to determine your strengths and weaknesses, and to identify how far your current score is from your score goal. If you have reviewed the MCAT topics covered in the earlier volumes of the **McGraw-Hill Education MCAT Test Preparation series**, you can use these tests to assess your mastery of the test content, to sharpen your test-taking skills, and to build your confidence for test day.

For best results, follow these four steps:

1. **Take each Practice Test under test conditions.** Find a quiet place where you will not be disturbed. Take the test as if it were the actual MCAT. Work through the test from beginning to end in one sitting. Mark your answers directly on the test pages. Observe the time limit given at the start of each section. If you have not finished a section when time runs out, mark the last question you answered and then note how much longer it takes you to complete the section. This information will tell you if you need to speed up your pace, and if so, by how much.

2. **Answer every question.** On the real MCAT, there is no penalty for wrong answers, so it makes sense to answer every question, even if you have to guess. If you don't know an answer, see if you can eliminate one or more of the answer choices. The more choices you can eliminate, the better your chance of guessing correctly!

3. **Check your answers in the Answer Explanations section at the end of the test.** Pay particular attention to the explanations for questions you missed.

4. **Fill out the Evaluation Charts.** A chart is located at the end of each Answer Explanations section. Mark the numbers of the questions you missed, and the chart will show you which sections of the companion volumes of the **MCAT Test Preparation Series** you still need to review.

MCAT

Practice Test 1

Biological and Biochemical Foundations of Living Systems

65 Questions   **Time Limit: 95 Minutes**

Questions 1–6 are based on the following passage.

Passage I

Leukemia is a term that describes a wide variety of blood cell cancers. Most leukemia cases involve elevated leukocyte counts. In acute cases of leukemia, immature leukocytes proliferate quickly, which leads to many abnormal immature cells in the bone marrow. This inhibits the ability of the bone marrow to produce healthy new leukocytes. This form of the cancer progresses rapidly, and the cells metastasize easily as they move into the bloodstream from the bone marrow. It can be fatal within weeks or months if not treated promptly. In contrast, chronic cases of leukemia typically involve the proliferation of abnormal mature leukocytes. This form of the disease progresses more slowly, and treatment need not always be immediate.

Once classified as acute or chronic, leukemia can be further subdivided into lymphocytic or myelogenous. This distinction depends on which type of leukocyte is abnormal in the patient. In lymphocytic leukemia, the lymphoid cells, such as the lymphocytes, are abnormal. In the myelogenous form, the myeloid cells, such as basophils, neutrophils, and eosinophils, are affected.

Chemotherapy drugs are often used in the management of leukemia cases. There are numerous categories of these drugs, and they have varied mechanisms of action. In treatment, several drugs are used in combination because some of the drugs are cell-cycle specific while others are not. Alkylating agents are capable of disrupting the function of DNA. Tubulin-binding agents are designed to interfere with microtubule formation. Other drugs are designed to interfere with DNA polymerase, DNA repair mechanisms, or protein synthesis or to act as purine analogs. Many of these drugs cannot enter into the brain when injected or ingested, so if the cancer has spread to this area, special methods must be used to introduce the drugs to the brain.

1. What would be the BEST explanation as to why people with chronic forms of leukemia can live longer untreated than those with acute cases of leukemia?
   A. Chronic cases involve types of leukocytes that have less important functions in the body.
   B. Chronic cases of leukemia involve abnormal cell division of mature cells, so there are still some immature cells that can proliferate into normal mature cells.
   C. The immune system is less likely to recognize and destroy abnormal immature leukocytes than it would be to recognize and destroy abnormal mature leukocytes.
   D. all of the above

2. What is the most logical explanation for why certain drugs may NOT be able to reach the brain if they have been ingested or injected?
   A. These drugs have a chemical nature that does not allow them to cross the blood-brain barrier.
   B. These drugs are so toxic that they are broken down before they reach the brain.
   C. Most of these drugs target only cancerous cells that normally would not be in the brain.
   D. The drugs that have been ingested have likely been denatured by the acids in the stomach.

3. A variety of risk factors exist for leukemia. Some of these factors include exposure to radiation, certain viral infections, and inherited tendencies. What do all of these factors have in common?
   A. All involve problems with protein translation in the cells.
   B. All can cause an increase in the production of cellular growth factors that enhance cell proliferation.
   C. All cause changes to the DNA that can lead to the production of altered proteins that can influence the development of cancer.
   D. All cause problems with transcription in the cells.

4. Many leukemia patients require antibiotic treatments frequently. Why would this be the case?
   A. Some antibiotics are known to be toxic to certain types of cancer cells and may help to damage the cancerous cells.
   B. The antibiotics might help to increase the function of the patient's immune system.
   C. The antibiotics can help prevent bacterial infections in the patient whose leukocyte function is compromised by the cancer.
   D. The antibiotics can help prevent viral infections in the patient.

5. Of the types of drugs mentioned in the passage, which category is most likely to be cell-cycle specific?
   A. tubulin-binding agents
   B. protein synthesis inhibitors
   C. purine analogs
   D. alkylating agents

6. It is not uncommon for leukemia patients to receive stem cell transplants. Why might this be a productive treatment option?
   A. The stem cells are capable of differentiating into new blood cells, which include the leukocytes, erythrocytes, and platelets.
   B. The stem cells can damage and replace the cancerous leukocytes.
   C. The stem cells can act as immune system modulators, enhancing the function of the entire system.
   D. The stem cells can temporarily replace the function of the cancerous cells and slow down the progression of the disease.

Questions 7–12 are based on the following passage.

Passage II

The kidneys are responsible for filtering certain components of blood and producing urine from them. In an adult, the kidneys are typically capable of processing about 1 to 1.5 liters of water per hour depending on the individual and conditions within the body. In a condition known as water intoxication, a person ingests more water (usually 3 or more liters in a single sitting) in a short period of time than the kidneys can process. In a child, the amount of water required to induce water intoxication is much less.

As the excess water moves from the digestive system, it accumulates in the plasma and extracellular fluids. Electrolytes such as sodium are drawn out of the cells in an attempt to equilibrate the concentrations inside and outside of the cells. As more and more water enters the extracellular fluids, the plasma sodium concentration drops, leading to a condition called *hyponatremia*, defined as a plasma sodium concentration less than 130 mmol/liter. Due to the effects of osmosis, water begins entering the cells. The cells will begin to swell and may eventually burst, if the condition is not reversed in a timely manner.

The situation becomes increasingly problematic as the cells and tissues of the central nervous system take in more water. Pressure builds in the brain that causes symptoms that resemble alcohol intoxication. Lightheadedness, nausea, vomiting, and headaches are typical as well. Damage can also occur to the lungs and heart. If not treated promptly, seizures, coma, and death can occur within several hours.

7. During water intoxication, the concentrations of the intracellular and extracellular fluids are not at equilibrium. In this situation, the extracellular fluid would be _____ to the cells.
   A. hypertonic
   B. isotonic
   C. hypotonic
   D. hyperosmotic

8. Imbalances in sodium ion concentrations would MOST likely cause problems with
   A. neuron function
   B. aerobic cellular respiration
   C. cell division
   D. muscle contraction

9. Of the options listed, what would be the best treatment for someone suffering from water intoxication?
   A. administering a saline solution that is more concentrated than the cells
   B. administering an isotonic solution
   C. administering a solution low in solute concentration
   D. performing dialysis to remove excess water from the plasma

10. Due to the excess water consumed that causes water intoxication, which of the following responses to this excess water would NOT be expected in the body?
    A. an increase in blood volume and pressure
    B. an increase in the secretion of antidiuretic hormone
    C. an increase in urine volume
    D. an increase in glomerular filtration rate

11. The regulation of water and sodium levels in the nephrons is adjusted in two regions of the kidneys where water and sodium can be reabsorbed from the nephron and returned to circulation. Those regions are the
    A. proximal convoluted tubule and distal convoluted tubule
    B. the loop of Henle and the distal convoluted tubule
    C. the distal convoluted tubule and the collecting duct
    D. the proximal convoluted tubule and the loop of Henle

12. Death that occurs due to water intoxication involves swelling and damage to certain parts of the central nervous system. Damage to which of these structures in the central nervous system would be MOST likely to have fatal consequences?
    A. the cerebrum
    B. the spinal cord
    C. the cerebellum
    D. the medulla oblongata

Questions 13–18 are based on the following passage.

Passage III

Sperm count in human males is influenced by a variety of factors. One of the most important variables affecting sperm count is the number of Sertoli cells located in seminiferous tubules of the testes. The Sertoli cells' primary function is to nurture cells through the process of spermatogenesis by providing them with nutrients and an environment conducive to spermatogenesis. Each Sertoli cell has a set number of spermatozoa that it can support. Sertoli cells have an additional role in forming the blood-testis barrier that provides immune privilege for the seminiferous tubules. This forms a physical barricade that keeps the developing sperm from coming into contact with cells of the immune system.

While it is not clear as to all the factors involved in determining Sertoli cell number, it is apparent that their development is most critical during the first nine months of life and prior to puberty. Events that affect the development of Sertoli cells in young males can influence fertility later in life. There may also be genetic factors involved in determining the number of Sertoli cells formed in a particular male.

The following data were collected from two groups of men. The men in group 1 had a normal sperm count while the men in group 2 were seeking infertility treatment due to a low sperm count. Levels of follicle stimulating hormone (FSH) and luteinizing hormone (LH) from the pituitary were measured as were the testicular hormones inhibin-B and testosterone in an attempt to determine which hormones seem to be linked to reduced sperm count.

Sample Group	LH	FSH	Inhibin-B	Testosterone
1	5.3 IU/L	5.0 IU/L	190 pg/mL	18.0 nmol/L
2	3.1 IU/L	17.6 IU/L	51 pg/mL	17.8 nmol/L

13. In which group would you expect to see a higher number of Sertoli cells?
    A. group 1
    B. group 2
    C. both groups 1 and 2
    D. impossible to tell from these data

14. Based on the data provided from both groups in the table, it is suggested that there is
    A. a positive feedback relationship between LH and FSH
    B. a negative feedback relationship between inhibin-B and FSH
    C. a positive feedback relationship between testosterone and FSH
    D. no relationship between these hormones

15. An elevated level of which hormone seems to be the best indicator of sperm count?
    A. LH
    B. FSH
    C. inhibin-B
    D. testosterone

16. Why would it be important for the Sertoli cells to establish a blood-testis barrier and immune privilege?
    A. to prevent the immune cells from attacking the sperm cells, which display different antigens from the other cells in the body
    B. to prevent the developing sperm cells from leaving the reproductive system
    C. to prevent blood from flowing into the testes
    D. to keep the developing sperm cells from entering into the epididymis before they are mature

17. The hormones FSH and LH are also involved in oogenesis in women. When LH surges in the ovarian cycle, what event will result?
    A. endometrium proliferation
    B. ovulation
    C. menstruation
    D. corpus luteum degradation

18. Fully differentiated Sertoli cells lose the ability to proliferate to produce more Sertoli cells. This would mean that they cannot perform
    A. mitosis
    B. meiosis
    C. apoptosis
    D. binary fission

Questions 19–24 are based on the following passage.

Passage IV

Evolutionary forces are capable of selecting for interesting traits within species. It is a generally accepted fact that testicle size in a variety of animals including primates is correlated with the reproductive behaviors of females within the species. In species where females are generally very promiscuous, male testes size is increased in relative proportion to their body weight. In species where females are monogamous with a single mate, the male testes size is decreased in proportion to body weight.

Recent studies have gone a step further and shown an interesting and somewhat controversial correlation between testicle size and brain size in 344 species of bats studied. The results suggested that there is an inverse relationship between the two. The data indicate that the bigger the testes size, the smaller the brain size. In bats, it seems that there is a tradeoff between the maintenance of brain mass and testicles.

Both tissues require an enormous energy investment to grow and maintain; therefore, the growth of one structure is at the sacrifice of the other. In bat species where the females are promiscuous, the testes size is large compared to the brain size. In those bat species were females are monogamous, the testes size is small compared to the brain size.

The following data represent brain and testes sizes as compared to body weight in three different species of bats:

Species	Brain Size (relative to body weight)	Testes Size (relative to body weight)
A	1.9%	8.0%
B	2.6%	1.3%
C	2.2%	2.1%

19. Based on the information in the passage, what might be the best explanation for the brain to testes size comparison for species C?
    A. Large testes size has been selected for by the females who are promiscuous and mate with many males.
    B. Large testes size has been selected against by the females who are monogamous and mate only with a single male.
    C. While the females of species C are not promiscuous, the females in this group may occasionally mate with more than one male, which is selecting for a slightly larger testes size.
    D. The majority of the energy is being spent on the maintenance of brain tissue leaving little energy left for maintenance of tissue in the testes.

20. In the data shown, species A has a testes size of 8% of its entire body weight. This might suggest that the testes in this species of bat have evolved to be huge in response to the reproductive behaviors of the female. Testes size of 8% of body weight is unheard of in primate species where the size of the testes never approaches 1% of body weight. Some critics of the bat study have suggested that it is not the testes size increasing in bat species A, but instead the overall body weight of this species of bat is decreasing. What evolutionary advantage would a decrease in body weight provide for this species of bat?
    A. It would allow for more energy to be focused on sperm production.
    B. Smaller bats are more likely to avoid predation.
    C. It would make the animal lighter, providing it with a flight advantage that would increase its endurance for food foraging while expending less energy than a larger bat.
    D. Smaller males are better able to mate with the females.

21. From an evolutionary perspective, why would it be appropriate for the male bats to make a tradeoff between testes size and brain size?

    A. Those males with large testes are more fit because they produce more sperm and are more likely to produce more offspring that share the same trait.

    B. Males with larger brains are more fit because they are more intelligent and can survive longer.

    C. Breeding behaviors must be learned in the bat population, and those with larger brains learn the breeding behaviors more quickly than those with smaller brains.

    D. all of the above

22. Primates vary greatly in their reproductive behaviors. Chimpanzees are prolific breeders and the females often mate with any male that they can find. Female gorillas typically breed only with the single alpha male of their social group, who spends much time defending his ranking. Hypothetically, which of the following would be expected if you were to extrapolate the results of the bat study to primates?

    A. Chimpanzees should have a large testes size and be less intelligent than gorillas.

    B. Gorillas should have large testes and be more intelligent than chimpanzees.

    C. Chimpanzees should have small testes and be more intelligent than gorillas.

    D. Gorillas should have small testes and be less intelligent than chimpanzees.

23. In a promiscuous population of bats, which individual would be considered most fit?

    A. the male that is largest and healthiest

    B. the individual with large testes who can produce enough sperm to reproduce often

    C. the female that is largest and healthiest

    D. the individual who has a large brain and can avoid predation well

24. The selection of males with large testes is an example of

    A. artificial selection

    B. stabilizing selection

    C. disruptive selection

    D. directional selection

Questions 25–30 are based on the following passage.

Passage V

Osteomyelitis is a bone infection often caused by the bacterium *Staphylococcus aureus,* which spreads through the blood to the bones. The infection is quite common after surgeries when soft tissues become infected and the infection moves to the adjacent bones. The long bones of children are particularly susceptible as they have excellent circulation to them during the growth period. In adults, the best circulation is to the vertebrae, and these are the bones that are most likely to develop osteomyelitis.

Osteomyelitis is treated with various antibiotics, but some patients have chronic infections that are not eradicated by antibiotic therapy due to a unique feature of *S. aureus*. *S. aureus* can be internalized by osteoblasts where the bacteria can continue to survive in the intracellular environment. Inside the osteoblasts, bacteria can induce apoptosis, killing their host cell. Surgical debridement is often required to remove the damaged and dead bone tissue created by the infection.

A major research question deals with how an *S. aureus* infection induces apoptosis in the host osteoblasts. In order for apoptosis to initiate in osteoblasts, the enzyme capsase-8 must be activated. This enzyme serves as a protease that cleaves critical proteins in the cell, causing cell death. Capsase-8 is only expressed under certain circumstances. In the case of osteomyelitis, the *S. aureus* bacteria cause the induction of tumor necrosis factor–related apoptosis-inducing ligand (TRAIL) in the osteoblasts. Then TRAIL activates capsase-8, which triggers a series of events leading to apoptosis and death of osteoblasts.

25. Which of the following potential drugs might be helpful in preventing the death of osteoblasts caused by *S. aureus* infection?
    A. one that increases capsase-8 activity
    B. one that increases TRAIL activity
    C. one that is an antagonist to TRAIL
    D. all of the above

26. Osteoblasts are unusual in that they actively engulf *S. aureus,* which survives in the osteoblast and eventually trigger apoptosis. In engulfing the bacteria, the osteoblasts resemble the normal activities of which type of leukocyte?
    A. basophils
    B. lymphocytes
    C. eosinophils
    D. macrophages

27. Osteomyelitis begins when *S. aureus* enters the bloodstream and moves to the bones. Under normal conditions, the nonspecific immune defense that would be activated as bacteria enter the blood would be
    A. antibody production by plasma cells
    B. cytotoxic T-cell activation
    C. the complement system
    D. interleukin secretion

28. Many strains of *S. aureus* that cause osteomyelitis are termed methicillin-resistant *Staphylococcus aureus* (MRSA). These strains have developed resistance to the antibiotic methicillin as well as to other antibiotics. The mechanism by which this antibiotic resistance occurs is by
    A. the overuse of antibiotics, which causes patients to become resistant to the antibiotics
    B. the overuse of antibiotics, which selects for bacteria that have mutations that allow them to survive in the presence of the antibiotics
    C. mutations, which occur as the bacteria are exposed to antibiotics that can serve as mutagens
    D. all of the above

29. The strains of *S. aureus* associated with osteomyelitis have a variety of cell adhesion molecules called *adhesins* that help them to attach to and be internalized by osteoblasts. These molecules are likely found in which of the following bacterial structures?
    A. the nucleoid
    B. the ribosomes
    C. the capsule
    D. spores

30. Osteoblasts are normally involved in building new bone matrix. Their activity is stimulated by the hormone _____ made by the _____.
    A. calcitonin; thyroid
    B. parathyroid hormone; parathyroid glands
    C. osteotonin; bone marrow
    D. none of the above

Questions 31–36 are based on the following passage.

Passage VI

Endothelin is a vasoactive peptide involved in a variety of processes, including the control of blood flow. Endothelin is capable of binding to two different receptors. There are receptors for endothelin located on smooth muscle (ETA) and receptors for endothelin located on vascular endothelium (ETB). When endothelin binds to ETA, it initiates vasoconstriction by narrowing blood vessels. However, when endothelin binds to ETB, vasodilation occurs due to the widening of blood vessels. The activity of the ETB receptor seems to counterregulate the ETA effects and prevents excessive vasoconstriction.

Drug X is a selective receptor antagonist for endothelin. It is designed to bind preferentially to certain endothelin receptors. Drug Y is another selective receptor antagonist for endothelin. It is also designed to preferentially bind to one of the endothelin receptors. Researchers are hopeful that drugs X and Y will be of value in the treatment of conditions such as pulmonary arterial hypertension (PAH). In PAH, excess endothelin is produced, which causes an increase in blood pressure within the pulmonary arteries. Normal pressure in the pulmonary arteries is expected to be about 14 mmHg, and pressure at or above 25 mmHg constitutes PAH. Both drugs have been tested in patients with PAH. There were five patients in each group. At the end of the study, the percent decrease in mean pulmonary artery pressure was measured for each patient and reported in the table.

Patient	Drug X	Drug Y	Placebo
1	+10%	−10%	+5%
2	+3%	−5%	0%
3	−5%	+2%	+13%
4	+2%	0%	−4%
5	0%	−7%	−2%
Average decrease	+2%	−4%	+2.4%

31. Based solely on the data provided, which conclusion should be drawn concerning the effectiveness of drugs X and Y?
    A. Drug X is a more effective treatment for PAH because most patients had a slight or no increase in pulmonary blood pressure while taking the drug.
    B. The placebo is the best treatment for PAH because some patients taking the placebo had a decrease in pulmonary blood pressure.
    C. Drugs X and Y should be used as combined therapy to maximize their effects.
    D. Drug Y is a more effective treatment for PAH because the majority of patients taking the drug had a decrease in pulmonary blood pressure.

32. Which endothelin receptor is drug X selectively binding to?
    A. ETA only
    B. ETB only
    C. both ETA and ETB
    D. neither ETA nor ETB

33. If a patient has PAH, the heart can become overly stressed and ultimately lead to heart failure. Which area of the heart is most likely to initially be affected by an increased blood pressure in the pulmonary arteries?
    A. the right and left atria
    B. the right and left ventricles
    C. the right ventricle
    D. the left ventricle

34. A patient overexpresses the ETB receptor. Explain what should happen to the patient's pressure.
    A. It should remain the same as long as the ETA receptor is also expressed.
    B. It should decrease due to elevated levels of vasodilation.
    C. It should increase since overexpression of ETB will block available ETA receptors.
    D. It should stay stable since other systems in the body will compensate.

35. Suppose a patient suffers from chronic systolic and diastolic hypertension due to an inherited defect in an endothelin receptor. How would the kidneys attempt to alleviate the hypertension?
    A. by decreasing water absorption in the nephrons
    B. by decreasing urine output thus increasing blood volume
    C. by increasing the amount of aldosterone secreted from the adrenal glands
    D. by increasing the amount of antidiuretic hormone secreted from the pituitary gland

36. In addition to regulation of vessel diameter, ETA is known to have other roles in the body. When activated by a specific type of endothelin, ETA can synergize with growth factors to cause rapid cell proliferation. Based on this information, it is most likely that ETA can be involved with
    A. an increase in metabolism
    B. the development of cancer
    C. immune system hypersensitivities
    D. increased stress to the kidneys and liver

Questions 37–42 are based on the following passage.

Passage VII

An endocrinologist has been studying an enzyme that she suspects is the rate-limiting step in the conversion of cholesterol to estrogen. It is reported in the literature that female mice with a mutation in the gene coding for this enzyme reach sexual maturity earlier than mice without the mutation. Controlled experiments are completed using breeding pairs of wild type mice and the mutant strain of mice. The plasma estrogen concentration is measured in female offspring at three weeks of age, prior to sexual maturity, which typically occurs by six weeks of age. The results, in estrogen pg/mL of plasma, are seen in the following table.

Trial	Wild Type	Mutant Strain
1	2.3	8.5
2	8.1	4.5
3	4.4	16.2
4	7.6	5.5
5	3.2	3.8
6	8.2	12.5
7	5.5	10.7
8	6.3	8.6

37. What conclusion can be made based on the data?
   A. The presence of the wild type enzyme increases estrogen concentration.
   B. The presence of the wild type enzyme increases cholesterol concentration.
   C. The presence of the mutant enzyme increases estrogen concentration.
   D. The presence of the mutant enzyme increases cholesterol concentration.

38. The rate-limiting step in a metabolic pathway
   A. requires the lowest activation energy
   B. is the fastest step in a metabolic pathway
   C. is always the last reaction in the pathway
   D. is the slowest step in a metabolic pathway

39. Recent studies have shown that cholesterol levels in women can vary significantly depending on where a woman is in her reproductive cycle. Most notable is the fact that total and LDL cholesterol levels typically decline at the points in the cycle where estrogen levels are at their highest. Based on this we would expect that total and LDL cholesterol levels would be the lowest
   A. following menopause
   B. during menstruation
   C. during ovulation
   D. prior to puberty

40. In addition to serving as a precursor for steroid biosynthesis, cholesterol has a variety of other roles in the body including
   A. maintenance of structural integrity and fluidity in plasma membranes
   B. nucleotide biosynthesis
   C. transport of molecules through the plasma membrane
   D. maintaining osmotic balance between cells and their surrounding environment

41. Based on the data presented, it is likely that
    A. wild type mice reach sexual maturity faster than the mutant strain
    B. the mutant strain mice will not reach sexual maturity
    C. the mutant strain mice have a lower cholesterol level than wild type mice
    D. wild type mice will not reach sexual maturity

42. If plasma cholesterol levels were to be measured, what would you expect to see in female mice that have reached sexual maturity as compared to female mice that are far from reaching sexual maturity?
    A. Cholesterol levels would be increased in wild type mice that have reached sexual maturity as compared to wild type mice that have not reached sexual maturity.
    B. Cholesterol levels would be the same in wild type mice that have reached sexual maturity as compared to wild type mice that have not reached sexual maturity.
    C. Cholesterol levels would be increased in mutant mice that have reached sexual maturity as compared to mutant mice that have not reached sexual maturity.
    D. Cholesterol levels would be decreased in mutant mice that have reached sexual maturity as compared to mutant mice that have not reached sexual maturity.

Questions 43–48 are based on the following passage.

Passage VIII

Human immunodeficiency virus (HIV) is known to infect T cells and macrophages possessing the CD4 receptor. In addition to the CD4 receptor, there are a variety of coreceptors that are also needed for certain strains of HIV to infect cells. One of these coreceptors is called CCR5 and is needed for the most common strains of HIV (called R5) to infect their host cells. The more CCR5 receptors a cell has, the greater the rate of infection for the cell. Some individuals have the delta-32 allele of CCR5 that leads to a decreased risk of HIV infection.

Women are at a much higher risk for contracting HIV from a male partner than a male is for contracting HIV from a female partner. Some of the increased risk for women is dependent on sex hormones. It has been hypothesized that women have different risks of contracting HIV at different points in their reproductive cycles. For example, women may be at a greater risk of contracting HIV following ovulation during the last two weeks of their cycle as opposed to the first two weeks of their cycle prior to ovulation. The difference between risk of infection before and after ovulation relates to sex hormones produced at various points in the reproductive cycle. It seems that the estrogen that is produced prior to ovulation provides a somewhat protective, although certainly not absolute, role against HIV infection. For women who do become infected with HIV, studies have shown that women in the first three to five years after HIV infection carry lower HIV viral loads than men, perhaps due to the influence of estrogen. This suggests a major role for sex hormones in the infection and progression of HIV.

43. According to the hypothesis presented concerning estrogen's role in HIV infection, which of these individuals would be at LEAST risk for HIV infection?
    A. a female producing elevated levels of testosterone
    B. a female with an ovarian tumor that causes increased secretion of estrogen
    C. a female who has had her ovaries removed
    D. a male with a reduced testosterone level

44. Women are at a higher risk of contracting HIV following ovulation. Based on the normal events of the female reproductive cycle, which hormone might account for the increased risk of HIV infection in women following ovulation?
    A. increased levels of progesterone
    B. increased levels of follicle stimulating hormone
    C. increased levels of estrogen
    D. increased levels of luteinizing hormone

45. As a result of chronic infection with HIV, the CCR5 gene is generally up-regulated over time. This would most likely account for
    A. an increased number of host cells becoming infected as the result of prolonged infection
    B. the elimination of HIV from the body in some individuals
    C. increased protection in women as the result of estrogen
    D. resistance of cells carrying the CCR5 receptor to infection

46. Some populations with the delta-32 CCR5 mutation seem to have close to 100% protection against HIV, while other populations with the delta-32 CCR5 mutation seem to have only partial protection. What could account for this difference?
    A. There is an environmental influence on expression of the delta-32 CCR5 phenotype.
    B. The delta-32 CCR5 allele exhibits incomplete dominance. Homozygotes have complete protection while heterozygotes have only partial protection.
    C. The expression of the delta-32 CCR5 allele can be masked by epistasis.
    D. Those that have only partial protection against HIV infection have been exposed to larger doses of HIV.

47. HIV belongs to a unique category of viruses termed retroviruses. Which of the following enzymes would be unique to retroviruses?
    A. DNA polymerase
    B. RNA polymerase
    C. reverse transcriptase
    D. helicase

48. Drugs such as AZT and ddI are nucleoside analogs used in HIV-infected patients. Both are chemically modified versions of the nucleotides that make up DNA and RNA. These modified nucleosides interfere with normal replication and transcription. The most important goal of these drugs would be
    A. to prevent the replication of host cell DNA so that the host cell cannot function
    B. to prevent the transcription of host cell RNA so that no proteins can be expressed
    C. to prevent the viral nucleic acid from entering the host cells
    D. to prevent replication of the viral genome

Questions 49–54 are based on the following passage.

Passage IX

In the past, there has been a great deal of controversy over the existence of viable but nonculturable (VBNC) states in bacteria. While normal culturing methods cannot detect these VBNC cells, there are a variety of molecular assays that can be used to indicate metabolic activity in the cells. Additionally, these cells can be resuscitated from VBNC states to a culturable state under appropriate conditions. The VBNC state has been observed in numerous species of bacteria and most recently in yeasts.

Escherichia coli is one of many species of bacteria that are able to enter and resuscitate from VBNC states. Certain strains of *E. coli* cause a variety of infections in humans. Urinary tract infections (UTIs) in women are frequently caused by *E. coli* that exist as harmless residents in the intestinal tract. These infections can be treated using antibiotics to kill the *E. coli*. However, about 30% of women treated for UTIs end up with a recurrence. For those who support the VBNC theory, it has been hypothesized that recurrent UTIs are caused by VBNC *E. coli* that resuscitate to initiate a new infection. These VBNC cells may not be killed using antibiotic therapies normally used to treat UTIs. Only culturable cells cause the symptoms of a UTI.

The following figure shows the number of *E. coli* bacteria present in a patient following antibiotic therapy for a UTI. Day 1 indicates the number of bacteria present at diagnosis. A urine sample was collected each day and cultured for the presence of *E. coli* as measured in colony forming units per milliliter of urine (cfu/ml). An assay was also used to determine the number of metabolically active cells that were potentially alive but not culturable (VBNC). The data are as follows:

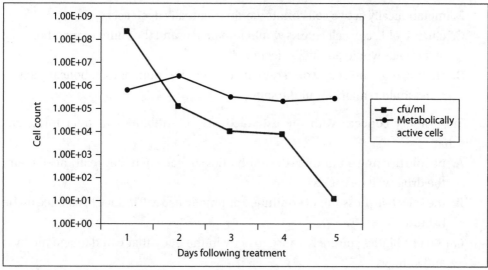

49. What can you conclude from the figure?
   A. Antibiotic therapy is highly effective at eliminating all *E. coli*.
   B. While the current infection has been effectively treated, this patient may be at risk for a recurrent UTI.
   C. The antibiotic therapy used for this patient was not sufficient to eliminate the infection.
   D. Antibiotic therapy has increased the total number of *E. coli* cells in this patient.

50. Which piece of information would be the BEST support for the existence of the VBNC state?
   A. the presence of DNA in the alleged VBNC cells
   B. the presence of an intact plasma membrane in the alleged VBNC cells
   C. the presence of specific proteins in the alleged VBNC cells
   D. the detection of transcription in the alleged VBNC cells

51. Why would women be more likely to contract a UTI caused by *E. coli* as compared to men?
   A. It is likely that the intestinal tracts of women contain a higher number of the *E. coli* bacteria as compared to men.
   B. The urethra of a female is closer to the intestinal tract than in a male, making it easier for the *E. coli* bacteria from the intestinal tract to gain access to the urinary tract.
   C. The *E. coli* bacteria in women are more likely to be resistant to antibiotic treatments.
   D. The immune system is less efficient in women, making infection more likely to occur.

52. If the antibiotic treatment used in the figure was continued for a period of 30 days, the most likely prediction would be that the
    A. cfu/mL of *E. coli* cell counts would begin to increase
    B. metabolically active cell counts would eventually decrease
    C. cfu/mL of *E. coli* cell counts would remain low and the count of metabolically active cells would gradually decrease
    D. cfu/mL of *E. coli* cells would remain low and the count of metabolically active cells would remain about the same

53. The primary concern with the extended use of antibiotics to treat infections is that
    A. people become immune to the antibiotics so that when they really need them, the drugs will be useless
    B. the selective pressures of continued antibiotic use will induce resistance in the bacteria
    C. the antibiotics routinely cause toxicity in the body that can damage the liver and kidneys
    D. the antibiotics encourage the overgrowth of resident bacteria in the body

54. One theory concerning VBNC cells is that they are simply on their way to dying. A piece of evidence that would refute that theory would be
    A. if some of the VBNC cells did die
    B. if the VBNC cells resuscitated
    C. if apoptosis was observed in the cells
    D. if no metabolic activity was observed

Questions 55–65 are not associated with a passage.

55. Which of the following explanations could account for the fact that dominant alleles that cause fatal disorders are less common than recessive alleles that cause fatal disorders?
    A. Every person carrying a single fatal dominant allele dies, whereas most individuals who carry a single recessive lethal allele live and reproduce.
    B. Recessive fatal alleles must cause sterility.
    C. Dominant alleles that cause fatal disorders are more serious than recessive lethal disorders.
    D. Dominant alleles are generally less common than recessive alleles.

56. A certain type of cell makes antibodies that are secreted from the cell. It is possible to track the path of these as they leave the cell by labeling them with radioactive isotopes. Which of the following might be the path of antibodies from where they are made to the cell membrane?
    A. Golgi complex to lysosomes to cell membrane
    B. rough endoplasmic reticulum to Golgi complex to cell membrane
    C. nucleus to Golgi complex to cell membrane
    D. smooth endoplasmic reticulum to lysosomes to cell membrane

57. A scientist suspects that the food in an ecosystem may have been contaminated with radioactive phosphates over a period of months. Which of the following substances could be examined for radioactive phosphate to test the hypothesis?
    A. the carbohydrates produced by plants in the area
    B. the DNA of the organisms in the area
    C. the lipids produced by organisms living in the area
    D. all of the above

58. Neurons contain a high concentration of potassium ions relative to the fluids surrounding them. How could a neuron acquire even more potassium?
    A. active transport
    B. osmosis
    C. endocytosis
    D. diffusion

59. At the end of the electron transport chain in aerobic cellular respiration, the final acceptor of the electrons is _____, which will then produce a molecule of _____.
    A. CO_2; O_2
    B. NAD^+; NADH
    C. O_2; H_2O
    D. ADP; ATP

60. A geneticist allows a cell to replicate in the presence of radioactive nucleotides. Which of the following would occur?
    A. The DNA in one of the daughter cells would be radioactive but not in the other daughter cell.
    B. The mRNA made by the daughter cells would be radioactive.
    C. The DNA in each of the daughter cells would be radioactive.
    D. The DNA would not be radioactive in either of the daughter cells.

61. How does DNA differ from RNA?
    A. DNA nucleotides use deoxyribose sugar; RNA uses ribose sugar.
    B. DNA uses the bases A, U, C, and G; RNA uses the bases A, T, C, and G.
    C. DNA is produced in transcription; RNA is produced in translation.
    D. RNA is a double-stranded molecule; DNA is a single-stranded molecule.

62. A human cell undergoes mitosis. Each of the resulting cells have _____ chromosomes.
    A. 8
    B. 23
    C. 46
    D. 92

63. When a nonsteroid (peptide) hormone binds to a receptor on the cell surface
    A. the hormone moves into the nucleus where it influences gene expression
    B. the hormone-receptor complex moves into the cytoplasm
    C. a second messenger will form within the cell
    D. the cell becomes inactive

64. The attachment site for RNA polymerase on the DNA template is called the
    A. promoter
    B. regulator
    C. operon
    D. repressor

65. Consider a bacterial cell that performs anaerobic respiration. If that bacterial cell had access to six molecules of glucose, how many molecules of ATP would it be able to produce?
    A. 2
    B. 6
    C. 12
    D. 36

STOP. This is the end of Section 1.

Chemical and Physical Foundations of Biological Systems

65 Questions   **Time Limit: 95 Minutes**

Questions 1–5 are based on the following passage.

Passage I

Many alkenes can be hydrated simply by treatment with a strong acid in the presence of water. The limitation of this method is that a carbocation is generated along the mechanistic pathway, opening the door to rearrangements, as shown in the sulfuric acid–catalyzed hydration of 3,3-dimethylbut-1-ene here:

One workaround for this problem is the oxymercuration-demercuration sequence, as shown here:

Consider the hydration of 3,6-dimethylcyclohex-1-ene under two separate conditions, for which four different alcohol products are proposed:

23

1. The most reasonable major hydration product of 3,6-dimethylcyclohex-1-ene using water and sulfuric acid is
   A. Product A
   B. Product B
   C. Product C
   D. Product D

2. The most reasonable major hydration product of 3,6-dimethylcyclohex-1-ene using oxymercuration-demercuration is
   A. Product A
   B. Product B
   C. Product C
   D. Product D

3. The structure giving six unique ^{13}C-NMR signals is most consistent with
   A. Product A
   B. Product B
   C. Product C
   D. Product D

4. Which of the following statements is MOST true for *trans*-3,6-dimethylcyclohex-1-ene?
   A. There are two chiral centers and the molecule is chiral.
   B. There are two chiral centers and the molecule is achiral.
   C. There are no chiral centers and the molecule is chiral.
   D. There are no chiral centers and the molecule is achiral.

5. The by-product of demercuration is
   A. Hg^0
   B. Hg^+
   C. Hg^{2+}
   D. Hg^{3+}

Questions 6–8 are not associated with a passage.

6. A peregrine falcon of 9 N is a bird known for its ability to reach extremely high speeds as it pursues prey. A bird in flight is subject to four forces: weight, drag, lift, and thrust. Which free body diagram accurately illustrates the direction of the forces acting on the bird assuming the bird is moving at constant velocity?

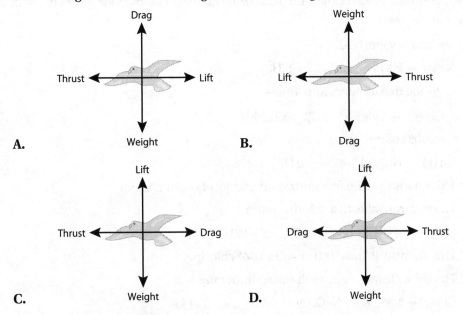

A.

B.

C.

D.

7. Blood is pumped from the heart at a rate of 5 L/min into the aorta of typical radius 1.2 cm. The velocity of blood as it enters the aorta is MOST nearly

   A. $9 \dfrac{\text{cm}}{\text{s}}$

   B. $12 \dfrac{\text{cm}}{\text{s}}$

   C. $18 \dfrac{\text{cm}}{\text{s}}$

   D. $32 \dfrac{\text{cm}}{\text{s}}$

8. In response to a heart attack, the normal heart rhythm is restored by a cardiac defibrillator, which transmits approximately 15 amperes of current through the chest during a time interval of 7 milliseconds. The amount of charge that flows during that time is

   A. 0.1 C
   B. 0.6 C
   C. 1.0 C
   D. 1.2 C

Questions 9–14 are based on the following passage.

Passage II

The reaction between sodium metal and chlorine gas is spontaneous and releases energy. The energy that is released is the enthalpy of formation of solid sodium chloride, which is also called the heat of formation. The reaction takes place in five elementary steps:

1. Sodium is vaporized.

    $Na\ (s) \rightarrow Na\ (g) \qquad \Delta H^o_{rxn} = 92\,kJ$

2. Chlorine decomposes into atoms.

    $\frac{1}{2}\,Cl_2\ (g) \rightarrow Cl\ (g) \qquad \Delta H^o_{rxn} = 121\,kJ$

3. Gaseous sodium atoms ionize.

    $Na\ (g) \rightarrow Na^+\ (g) + e^- \qquad \Delta H^o_{rxn} = 496\,kJ$

    This quantity is the first ionization energy of sodium vapor.

4. The electron adds to a chlorine atom.

    $Cl\ (g) + e^- \rightarrow Cl^-\ (g) \qquad \Delta H^o_{rxn} = -349\,kJ$

    This quantity is the electron affinity of chlorine.

5. The chloride ion reacts with the sodium ion.

    $Cl^-\ (g) + Na^+\ (g) \rightarrow NaCl\ (s) \qquad \Delta H^o_{rxn} = -771\,kJ$

Addition of the five elementary equations gives the sum equation for the formation of solid sodium chloride. Most of the energy that is given off is due to the formation of solid sodium chloride from the gaseous ions. In solid sodium chloride, each positive ion is surrounded by six negative ions, and each negative ion is surrounded by six positive ions in a cubic lattice array. The lattice energy of an ionic compound is a measure of the attractive forces between the ions. The higher the lattice energy, the stronger the attractions and the higher melting the solid. Lattice energies depend on the charge and on the size of the ions in the array. If the size is constant, increasing charge increases the lattice energy. If the charge is constant, increasing size lowers the lattice energy.

Some lattice energies are given in the table.

Compound	Lattice Energy in kJ/mole
LiCl	834
KCl	701
Na_2O	2481
MgO	3795
Na_2S	2192

9. When one mole of sodium metal reacts with one mole of chlorine gas to form solid sodium chloride, what is the heat of formation?
   A. $-771 \, kJ$
   B. $+771 \, kJ$
   C. $-411 \, kJ$
   D. $+411 \, kJ$

10. What is the electron configuration of chloride?
    A. $1s^2 2s^2 2p^6 3s^2 3p^5$
    B. $1s^2 2s^2 2p^6 3s^2 3p^6$
    C. $1s^2 2s^2 2p^6 3s^2 3p^6 4s^1$
    D. $1s^2 2s^2 2p^6 3s^2 3p^6 3d^1$

11. Why is the lattice energy of Na_2S so much greater than that of NaCl?
    A. Two sodium ions are needed for every sulfide.
    B. Sulfide has a greater charge than chloride and is about the same size.
    C. Sulfide is much smaller than chloride.
    D. Chloride has a negative one charge, whereas sulfide has a negative two charge.

12. Which of the following represents the lattice energy of sodium chloride?
    A. $+771 \, kJ$
    B. $-771 \, kJ$
    C. $+411 \, kJ$
    D. $-411 \, kJ$

13. Which Lewis dot structure BEST represents the sodium ion?
    A. Na
    B. Na$^\bullet$
    C. Na$^+$
    D. Na$^-$

14. The reaction of chlorine gas and sodium metal also produces light. How is the light produced?
    A. The electrons absorb heat energy and release it as light.
    B. Light is emitted when the electrons become gaseous.
    C. Light is emitted when the metal atom becomes gaseous.
    D. Light is emitted when the chlorine becomes atomic.

Questions 15–19 are based on the following passage.

Passage III

Image formation in the human eyeball occurs when parallel light rays refract through the eye lens and converge on the retina. Hyperopia, or farsightedness, is a common vision problem that occurs as a result of these light rays entering the eyeball but converging behind the cornea. This results in the ability to see distant objects clearly with vision becoming blurry for close objects. Hyperopia, as is the case with many vision problems, can generally be corrected with eyeglass lenses, specifically a converging lens, as shown in the figure. A converging lens positioned in front of a hyperopic eye acts to focus the light rays sooner so that they converge on the retina rather than behind the retina.

Correction of hyperopia is accomplished with a converging lens tailored to characteristics unique to the person. The following table lists four different scenarios of a converging lens, with each scenario detailing the distance of an identical object placed in front of the same converging lens as well as the focal length of the lens.

Characteristics of a Converging Eyeglass Lens		
Converging Lens Scenario	**Object Distance (p) (cm)**	**Focal Length (f) (cm)**
1	3f	f
2	2f	f
3	f	f
4	$\dfrac{f}{2}$	f

15. Which converging lens scenario will NOT produce an image?
    A. Lens Scenario 1
    B. Lens Scenario 2
    C. Lens Scenario 3
    D. Lens Scenario 4

16. Which converging lens scenario will produce an image that is virtual and upright?
    A. Lens Scenario 1
    B. Lens Scenario 2
    C. Lens Scenario 3
    D. Lens Scenario 4

17. The image distance for Lens Scenario 2 is
    A. 3f
    B. between 2f and 3f
    C. 2f
    D. f

18. The magnification of the image for Lens Scenario 1 indicates that, with respect to the object, the image
    A. is reduced by 2
    B. remains the same
    C. is enlarged by 2
    D. is enlarged by 3

19. The focal length is related to the object distance and the image distance according to:
    A. $\dfrac{(\text{object distance})(\text{image distance})}{\text{image distance} + \text{object distance}}$

    B. $\dfrac{(\text{object distance})(\text{image distance})}{\text{image distance} - \text{object distance}}$

    C. $\dfrac{\text{image distance} + \text{object distance}}{(\text{object distance})(\text{image distance})}$

    D. $\dfrac{\text{image distance} - \text{object distance}}{(\text{object distance})(\text{image distance})}$

Questions 20–22 are not associated with a passage.

20. Which of the following Fischer projections MOST accurately describes the boxed molecule?

optically pure

A.
```
      Me
  Br ──┼── H
  Br ──┼── H
      Me
```

B.
```
      Me
  Br ──┼── H
  H  ──┼── Br
      Me
```

C.
```
      Me
  H  ──┼── Br
  Br ──┼── H
      Me
```

D.
```
      Me
  H  ──┼── Br
  H  ──┼── Br
      Me
```

21. For the following reaction, the most reasonable starting material is

$$? \xrightarrow[\substack{H_2SO_4 \\ H_2O}]{K_2Cr_4O_7} \xrightarrow[Et_2O]{CH_2N_2}$$

(product: structure with Ph and CO_2Me, *optically pure*)

A. Ph / OH

B. Ph / OH

C. Ph / OH

D. Ph / OH

22. For the following reaction, the most likely product is a(n)

(structure with Cl, *optically pure*) $\xrightarrow[THF]{t\text{-BuOK}}$?

A. ether with optical activity
B. ether without optical activity
C. alkene with optical activity
D. alkene without optical activity

Questions 23–27 are based on the following passage.

Passage IV

An important class of oxidation-reduction reactions is called single displacement. In single displacement reactions, one element takes the place of another in a compound. The reactivity series for metals is a summary of the results of many single displacement experiments. A metal that is above another is more reactive and will take the place of the lower, less reactive metal in a compound.

For instance, a student places a sample of zinc metal into a solution of nickel (II) nitrate. The zinc reacts to displace the nickel ions as follows:

$$Zn \ (s) + Ni(NO_3)_2 \ (aq) \rightarrow Ni \ (s) + Zn(NO_3)_2 \ (aq)$$

The reactivity series also predicts the reactivity of a metal with water. Only a few metals—the Group I metals and calcium, strontium, and barium from Group II—react with water at room temperature. This reaction is similar to a single displacement because the metal displaces the hydrogen in water. It is often called a hydrogen displacement reaction.

Dilute acid, usually hydrochloric acid, can be used to compare the reactivity of metals that do not react with water.

Experiment

A student reacts samples of copper, cobalt, and iron metal with dilute hydrochloric acid with the following results:

Metal	Reaction with HCl
Cu	No reaction
Co	Slow reaction with formation of small bubbles
Fe	Rapid reaction with formation of large bubbles

Activity Series
K Na Ca Mg Al Mn Zn Cr Fe Ni Sn Pb Cu Ag Au
Better Reducing Agent   **Better Oxidizing Agent**

A general rule for the main group metals is that the reactivity of metals within a group increases going down the column, and the reactivity decreases going from left to right across a row. For transition metals, the reactivity does not change in a regular manner across a row but does decrease going down a column.

23. Which of the following BEST represents the reaction of calcium with water?

   A. $Ca\ (s) + H_2O\ (l) \rightarrow CaOH\ (s) + H\ (g)$

   B. $Ca\ (s) + H_2O\ (l) \rightarrow Ca(OH)_2\ (s) + H_2\ (g)$

   C. $Ca\ (s) + 2H_2O\ (l) \rightarrow Ca(OH)_2\ (s) + H_2\ (g)$

   D. $Ca^{+2}\ (aq) + 2H_2O\ (l) \rightarrow Ca(OH)_2\ (aq) + H_2\ (g)$

24. Which of the following is the first metal in the activity series that does NOT react with water?

   A. Mg

   B. Al

   C. Mn

   D. Zn

25. Where would cobalt be expected to fall in the activity series?

   A. between lead and copper

   B. to the left of iron

   C. between iron and copper

   D. to the right of copper

26. Which of the following statements is NOT true?
    A. Nickel will displace silver from silver (I) nitrate.
    B. Chromium reacts with dilute hydrochloric acid.
    C. Calcium will displace aluminum from aluminum nitrate.
    D. Tin will displace nickel from nickel (II) nitrate.

27. What is the electron configuration of chromium?
    A. $[Ar]4s^2 3d^4$
    B. $[Ar]3d^5 4s^1$
    C. $[Ne]3d^5 4s^1$
    D. $[Ar]4s^0 3d^6$

Questions 28–30 are not associated with a passage.

28. Which of the following metals is diamagnetic?
    A. Calcium
    B. Aluminum
    C. Titanium
    D. Copper

29. Iodine-131, a radioisotope typically employed in the diagnosis of thyroid disorders, has a mass number, A, of 131 and an atomic number, Z, of 53. The number of neutrons, N, of iodine-131 is
    A. 131
    B. 78
    C. 53
    D. 25

30. Ten milliliters of blood is drawn for routine testing. Assuming the density of human blood is $1.06\,g/cm^3$, the weight of the blood sample is
    A. 0.1 N
    B. 1.0 N
    C. 10.0 N
    D. 20.0 N

Questions 31–35 are based on the following passage.

Passage V

The $S_N 2$ reaction is applicable to a wide variety of substrates, and it is impacted by many parameters. First, a good leaving group is required for $S_N 2$ to take place. Second, nucleophilic displacement is dependent upon a strong nucleophile; however, most potential nucleophiles exhibit both basic and nucleophilic character. As nucleophiles become more basic, the competing pathway of bimolecular elimination (E2) begins to predominate.

boron 5 **B** 10.811	carbon 6 **C** 12.011	nitrogen 7 **N** 14.007	oxygen 8 **O** 15.999	fluorine 9 **F** 18.998
aluminium 13 **Al** 26.982	silicon 14 **Si** 28.086	phosphorus 15 **P** 30.974	sulfur 16 **S** 32.065	chlorine 17 **Cl** 35.453
			selenium 34 **Se** 78.96	bromine 35 **Br** 79.904
				iodine 53 **I** 126.90

Two more parameters also exert influence on reactivity: the electrophilic center (i.e., primary, secondary, or tertiary) and the solvent (i.e., nonpolar, polar protic, or polar aprotic). A student mixes equimolar quantities of 2-chloropropane, 2-iodopropane, sodium methoxide (NaOMe), and sodium methyl thiolate (NaSMe) in a solvent of methanol, and observes both S_N2 and E2 reactivity.

31. In comparing methoxide (MeO^-) and methyl thiolate (MeS^-), methoxide is
    A. more nucleophilic and more basic
    B. more nucleophilic and less basic
    C. less nucleophilic and more basic
    D. less nucleophilic and less basic

32. In comparing chloride (Cl^-) and iodide (I^-), chloride is
    A. the better leaving group and the better nucleophile
    B. the better leaving group and the poorer nucleophile
    C. the poorer leaving group and the better nucleophile
    D. the poorer leaving group and the poorer nucleophile

33. The fastest S_N2 reaction would occur between
    A. methoxide and 2-iodopropane
    B. methoxide and 2-chloropropane
    C. methyl thiolate and 2-iodopropane
    D. methyl thiolate and 2-chloropropane

34. If temperature is increased,
    A. the rate of E2 increases; the rate of S_N2 decreases
    B. the rate of S_N2 increases; the rate of E2 decreases
    C. the rate of both reactions increases
    D. the rate of both reactions decreases

35. Which of the following solvents would provide for the fastest S_N2 reaction?
    A. Methanol
    B. Dimethylsulfoxide
    C. Tetrahydrofuran
    D. Diethyl ether

Questions 36–42 are based on the following passage.

Passage VI

Cervical traction devices employ forces transmitted through a system of pulleys to correct deformities of the neck and spine by maintaining their proper alignment. The physics involved in these devices are based on Newton's second law of motion and Atwood's machine.

Newton's second law of motion states that a net force, F_{net}, acting in a given direction on an object of mass, m, will result in an acceleration, a, of the object in that same direction, i.e.:

$$\sum F = ma$$

or

$$\sum F_x = ma_x \text{ and } \sum F_y = ma_y$$

Atwood's machine, illustrated in the following figure, uses a block-and-pulley system to determine the acceleration of the system as well as other variables such as the falling distance of either mass and the tension in the string connecting the masses.

In a typical experimental setup, the Atwood machine is assembled with a massless string around a pulley. Connected on either end of the string are two masses, m_1 and m_2, where $m_1 \neq m_2$. The pulley is considered to be massless as well as frictionless. When the connected masses are released, both masses will accelerate at the same rate with the larger mass accelerating downward and the smaller mass accelerating upward.

Students were asked to conduct experiments using Atwood's machine with a constant total mass of 300 g. They were given hanging weights in increments of 10 g and could place any number of weights on either side of Atwood's machine as long as the total mass equaled 300 g.

36. For a typical Atwood's machine setup, the free-body diagram of the side with m_1 is

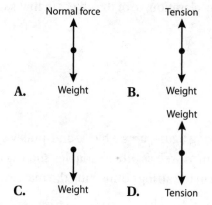

37. A general expression for the acceleration of the system in Atwood's machine is

A. $a = \dfrac{(m_2 - m_1)}{(m_1 + m_2)} g$

B. $a = \dfrac{(m_2 + m_1)}{(m_1 + m_2)} g$

C. $a = \dfrac{(m_2 \cdot m_1)}{(m_1 + m_2)} g$

D. $a = \dfrac{(m_2)}{(m_1 + m_2)} g$

38. A trial is conducted using the Atwood's machine with $m_1 = 140\,g$ and $m_2 = 160\,g$. The tension in the string is approximately

A. 0.8 N

B. 1.2 N

C. 1.5 N

D. 1.9 N

39. Students applied masses to the Atwood's machine setup such that $m_1 = 80\,g$ and $m_2 = 220\,g$. The acceleration of the system is

A. $1.7\,\dfrac{m}{s^2}$

B. $2.4\,\dfrac{m}{s^2}$

C. $3.3\,\dfrac{m}{s^2}$

D. $4.6\,\dfrac{m}{s^2}$

40. In an experimental trial in which the students used masses $m_1 = 110\,g$ and $m_2 = 190\,g$, they were asked to determine the tension in the string, which they found to be

A. 1.4 N

B. 1.9 N

C. 2.8 N

D. 3.3 N

41. An assumption of the calculation for the acceleration of the system of masses in Atwood's machine is that the pulley is frictionless. If one uses a pulley with friction, the expression for the acceleration of the system now becomes

   A. $a = \dfrac{m_2 g - m_1 g - f}{(m_1 + m_2)}$

   B. $a = \dfrac{m_1 g - m_2 g - f}{(m_1 + m_2)}$

   C. $a = \dfrac{-f}{(m_1 + m_2)}$

   D. $a = \dfrac{(m_1 + m_2)}{m_2 g - m_1 g - f}$

42. In an experiment using a pulley with friction, the students collect data and create a graph of acceleration versus mass difference. From the graph, the students can determine the frictional force from the
   A. x-variable
   B. y-variable
   C. slope
   D. y-intercept

Questions 43–47 are based on the following passage.

Passage VII

The Jones oxidation is a classical methodology for the oxidation of secondary alcohols to ketones. The conditions involve the combination of potassium dichromate ($K_2Cr_2O_7$), a shelf-stable crystalline solid, and aqueous sulfuric acid (H_2SO_4). This is simply a way to produce chromic acid (H_2CrO_4) in situ:

$$KO-\overset{\overset{\displaystyle O}{\|}}{\underset{\underset{\displaystyle O}{\|}}{Cr}}-O-\overset{\overset{\displaystyle O}{\|}}{\underset{\underset{\displaystyle O}{\|}}{Cr}}-OK \quad \xrightarrow[H_2O]{H_2SO_4} \quad 2\,HO-\overset{\overset{\displaystyle O}{\|}}{\underset{\underset{\displaystyle O}{\|}}{Cr}}-OH$$

   Under the reaction conditions, chromic acid produces equilibrium concentrations of chromium trioxide (CrO_3), which is the key oxidizing agent in the Jones oxidation:

$$HO-\overset{\overset{\displaystyle O}{\|}}{\underset{\underset{\displaystyle O}{\|}}{Cr}}-OH \quad \underset{}{\overset{H^+}{\rightleftharpoons}} \quad O{=}\overset{\overset{\displaystyle O}{\|}}{Cr}{\scriptstyle\diagdown}O \quad + \quad H_2O$$

Chromium trioxide reacts with alcohols to provide chromate esters, which proceeds as follows:

With primary alcohols, however, the reaction does not stop at the aldehyde stage. In the presence of acid and water, the initially formed carbonyl compounds are in equilibrium with their hydrates:

The hydrates can form chromate esters with one of the hydroxyl groups, just as the alcohol substrates do. When R′ = H, this proton is easily lost to provide the carboxylic acid. Therefore, under Jones conditions, secondary alcohols yield ketones, but primary alcohols give carboxylic acids:

If aldehydes are desired from primary alcohols, the oxidation can be carried out with pyridinium chlorochromate (PCC), a shelf-stable crystalline solid that also provides chromium trioxide:

pyridinium chlorochromate
(PCC)

43. Ketones are NOT oxidized to carboxylic acids under Jones conditions because
    A. they do not form hydrates with water
    B. their hydrates cannot form chromate esters
    C. the chromate esters of their hydrates cannot decompose by proton loss
    D. the chromate ester decomposition is reversible

44. Pyridinium chlorochromate (PCC) is selective for the production of aldehydes from primary alcohols because
    A. it can be weighed out very accurately
    B. it does not introduce water into the reaction
    C. the pyridine prevents overoxidation
    D. the environment is less acidic

45. Consider the Jones oxidation of heptane-1,6-diol:

The most likely product of this reaction would be a(n)
   A. hydroxy ketone
   B. hydroxy acid
   C. oxo aldehyde
   D. oxo acid

46. Consider the PCC oxidation of heptane-1,6-diol:

The most likely product of this reaction would be
   A. a hydroxy ketone
   B. a hydroxy acid
   C. oxo aldehyde
   D. an oxo acid

47. A tertiary alcohol is treated with the Jones reagent, and the reaction mixture is worked up and purified. The most likely compound isolated is
   A. an alcohol
   B. a ketone
   C. an aldehyde
   D. a carboxylic acid

Questions 48–52 are based on the following passage.

Passage VIII

α-D-Glucose and β-D-glucose are interconverted through a process known as mutarotation, which proceeds via a ring-opened intermediate, as shown:

In solution, α-D-glucose and β-D-glucose exist in a 9:16 ratio at equilibrium, but this is not what would be predicted from sterics alone. The discrepancy is largely due to the anomeric effect, which involves the interaction of the lone pairs on the ring oxygen with the C-1 hydroxy group.

48. The best term for describing the difference between α-D-glucose and β-D-glucose is
    A. enantiomers
    B. diastereomers
    C. regioisomers
    D. conformers

49. Aside from the multiple alcohols, the functional group found in both α-D-glucose and β-D-glucose is a(n)
    A. hemiacetal
    B. acetal
    C. aminal
    D. orthoester

50. Aside from the multiple alcohols, the functional group found in the ring-opened intermediate is a(n)
    A. ketone
    B. aldehyde
    C. acid
    D. ester

51. α-D-Glucose and β-D-glucose are BEST described as
    A. hexoses and furanoses
    B. pentoses and furanoses
    C. hexoses and pyranoses
    D. pentoses and pyranoses

52. The BEST rationale for the impact of the anomeric effect on the equilibrium of α-D-glucose and β-D-glucose is
    A. it stabilizes α-D-glucose and destabilizes β-D-glucose
    B. it destabilizes α-D-glucose and stabilizes β-D-glucose
    C. it stabilizes both α-D-glucose and β-D-glucose
    D. it destabilizes both α-D-glucose and β-D-glucose

Questions 53–57 are based on the following passage.

Passage IX

In the general chemistry laboratory, it is convenient to carry out most reactions in solution, usually aqueous solution. When solid ionic compounds are mixed together at room temperature, no reaction takes place. But if aqueous solutions of the solids are mixed, a reaction can take place. Common types of reactions in aqueous solution include acid-base reactions, precipitation reactions, and oxidation-reduction reactions.

Compounds have different solubilities in water, as shown in the following table:

Solubilities of Some Substances		
Compound	Temp (°C)	Solubility (g/100 mL water)
NaCl (s)	0	35.7
NaCl (s)	100	39.1
$PbCl_2$ (s)	20	0.99
$PbCl_2$ (s)	100	3.34
AgCl (s)	10	0.000089
AgCl (s)	100	0.0021
CH_3CH_2OH (l)	20	∞
$CH_3CH_2OCH_2CH_3$ (l)	15	8.43

Ions in water solution are called electrolytes, and a solution of electrolytes will conduct electricity. The ability to conduct electricity is called conductivity, and it is directly related to the concentration of ions in solution. Ionic compounds that are very soluble in water are strong electrolytes. Ionic compounds that are sparingly soluble in water are weak electrolytes. Covalent compounds can be strong, weak, or even nonelectrolytes. It depends on whether the substance can form ions in solution, and if so, the concentration of the ions.

A general rule for predicting whether a reaction will take place when two electrolytic solutions are mixed is that a reaction will take place if one or both possible products are either insoluble, weak, or nonelectrolyte.

Experiment

A student determines if each of a series of compounds was soluble or insoluble in water. The results are as follows.

Compound	Soluble in Water
NaCl	yes
$NaNO_3$	yes
$AgNO_3$	yes
$BaSO_4$	no
$Ba(NO_3)_2$	yes
Na_2SO_4	yes
NaOH	yes
$Ca(OH)_2$	no
Na_3PO_4	yes
$Ca_3(PO_4)_2$	no

53. What is the expected insoluble product when a solution of silver nitrate reacts with a solution of sodium chloride at room temperature?
    A. sodium nitrate
    B. silver nitrate
    C. silver chloride
    D. sodium chloride

54. A student prepares a saturated solution of sodium chloride at 100.0°C. The student makes 250.0 mL of solution and then cools it to 0.0°C. How many grams of NaCl will precipitate out when the solution is cooled to 0.0°C?
    A. 89.3 g
    B. 97.8 g
    C. 8.6 g
    D. 3.4 g

55. What would happen to the conductivity of a mixture of two solutions that produces two insoluble products?
    A. It would remain the same.
    B. It would lessen somewhat.
    C. It would decrease greatly.
    D. It would increase greatly.

56. Which of the following statements can BEST be inferred from the experimental results?
    A. Sodium salts are always soluble.
    B. Group II salts are always soluble.
    C. Phosphates are usually insoluble.
    D. Sulfates are usually soluble.

57. Based on the experimental data, which of the following statements is true?
    A. Silver compounds are always insoluble.
    B. Phosphates are always insoluble.
    C. Sulfates are never soluble.
    D. You can improve the solubility of silver chloride with the addition of ammonia.

Question 58 is not associated with a passage.

58. Which of the following shows a pair of substances that differ from the other three?
    A. NH_4^+ and NH_3
    B. H_2SO_4 and SO_4^{2-}
    C. $H_2PO_4^-$ and HPO_4^{2-}
    D. HCl and Cl^-

Questions 59–63 are based on the following passage.

Passage X

Human tooth enamel is composed of the mineral hydroxyapatite, which has the formula $Ca_5(PO_4)_3OH$. It is insoluble in water, but due to its basicity, it is soluble in acid solution.

Plaque forms on teeth due to a combination of carbohydrates and proteins, called mucin, which produces a film that builds up if not removed by thorough cleaning of the teeth and gums. Plaque traps food particles, which can be fermented by bacteria and produce lactic acid. Saliva does contain buffering agents that can neutralize acid in the mouth, but saliva cannot penetrate solid plaque. Lactic acid levels can drop to as low as pH 4.5 inside the plaque. As the plaque becomes more acidic, hydroxyapatite is converted to calcium hydrogen phosphate, which dissolves in water. The equation is as follows:

$$Ca_5(PO_4)_3OH \text{ (s)} + 4\,H_3O^+ \text{ (aq)} \rightarrow 3\,CaHPO_4 \text{ (aq)} + 2\,Ca^{+2} \text{ (aq)} + 5\,H_2O \text{ (l)}$$

When the hydroxyapatite reacts, cavities can form. The addition of fluoride to municipal water supplies and to toothpaste has lowered the incidence of cavities in children in the United States. Many children also have fluoride treatments as part of their routine dental care.

Fluoride has the ability to replace the hydroxide ion in hydroxyapatite, forming a compound called fluoroapatite. Fluoroapatite not only has a smaller K_{sp} value than hydroxyapatite, it is less basic as well. Thus it is far less soluble in acid solution. The reaction of fluoride with hydroxyapatite is as follows:

$$Ca_5(PO_4)_3OH \text{ (s)} + F^- \text{ (aq)} \rightleftharpoons Ca_5(PO_4)_3F \text{ (s)} + OH^- \text{ (aq)}$$

The K_{sp} of hydroxyapatite is 7×10^{-37}. The K_{sp} of fluoroapatite is 1×10^{-60}.

59. The dissolution of hydroxyapatite in water is BEST represented by

    A. $Ca_5(PO_4)_3OH \text{ (s)} \rightleftharpoons 5\,Ca \text{ (aq)} + 3\,PO_4 \text{ (aq)} + OH \text{ (aq)}$

    B. $Ca_5(PO_4)_3OH \text{ (s)} \rightleftharpoons Ca_5 \text{ (aq)} + (PO_4)_3 \text{ (aq)} + OH \text{ (aq)}$

    C. $Ca_5(PO_4)_3OH \text{ (s)} \rightleftharpoons Ca_5 \,(PO_4)_3^{+1} \text{ (aq)} + OH^- \text{ (aq)}$

    D. $Ca_5(PO_4)_3OH \text{ (s)} \rightleftharpoons 5\,Ca^{+2} \text{ (aq)} + 3\,PO_4^{-3} \text{ (aq)} + OH^- \text{ (aq)}$

60. Why does the equilibrium of the reaction of hydroxyapatite with fluoride lie to the right?

    A. Fluoride is a weaker base than hydroxide.

    B. Hydroxide can be removed as it is formed by buffers in saliva.

    C. Fluoroapatite is less soluble than the reactant.

    D. The product solidifies onto the surface of the tooth.

61. A larger K_{sp} value means that
    A. reactants predominate
    B. products predominate
    C. there is a lower concentration of ions
    D. the solid is less soluble

62. What is the effect on the solubility of hydroxyapatite if calcium ions are added to a saturated solution?
    A. The equilibrium will shift to the right.
    B. The equilibrium will shift to the left.
    C. There will be no effect.
    D. More hydroxyapatite will ionize.

63. The solubility of hydroxyapatite, x, can be found from
    A. $K_{sp} = x^3$
    B. $K_{sp} = x^5$
    C. $K_{sp} = x^7$
    D. $K_{sp} = x^9$

Questions 64 and 65 are not associated with a passage.

64. Which of the following represents the proper Lewis structure for fluoride?
    A. $:\overset{\cdot\cdot}{\underset{\cdot\cdot}{F}}\cdot$
    B. $:\overset{\cdot\cdot}{\underset{\cdot\cdot}{F}}:$
    C. $:\overset{\cdot\cdot}{\underset{\cdot\cdot}{F}}:^+$
    D. $:\overset{\cdot\cdot}{\underset{\cdot\cdot}{F}}:^-$

65. Under normal conditions, blood is pumped from the heart into the circulatory system under a systolic pressure of 120 mmHg (*note*: 1 mmHg = 1333 N/m^2). Assuming the diameter of the aorta is 3.0 cm, the force exerted by the beating heart on the blood as it enters the circulatory system is approximately
    A. 31 N
    B. 68 N
    C. 95 N
    D. 114 N

STOP. This is the end of Section 2.

Psychological, Social, and Biological Foundations of Behavior

65 Questions   **Time Limit: 95 Minutes**

Questions 1–5 are not associated with any passage.

1. Alfred is looking through a telescope with one eye closed watching sailboats enter a harbor. He is able to tell that a 20-foot boat has entered before a 30-foot catamaran. Which of the following cues is Alfred NOT able to use to judge relative distance?
   A. relative size
   B. interposition
   C. retinal disparity
   D. texture

2. With which theoretical paradigm is the German political philosopher Karl Marx most associated?
   A. conflict theory
   B. functionalism
   C. symbolic interactionism
   D. avoidance theory

3. According to the bystander effect, which is MOST likely to be true in an emergency?
   A. the greater the number of people present, the slower the response because of increased diffusion of responsibility
   B. the greater the number of people present, the slower the response because of decreased diffusion of responsibility
   C. the greater the number of people present, the faster the response because of increased diffusion of responsibility
   D. the greater the number of people present, the faster the response because of decreased diffusion of responsibility

4. Which theoretical paradigm sees aspects of society as separate but interrelated, with each component acting separately but critical to the functioning of the whole?
   A. functionalism
   B. conflict theory
   C. symbolic interactionism
   D. societal relativism

5. Studies examining altruism have shown that which of the following is true?
   A. True altruism is common and found even between highly disparate individuals.
   B. Altruism is more frequent in larger communities due to diffusion of responsibility.
   C. Altruism is more likely to occur between individuals who are likely to reciprocate assistance in the future.
   D. Altruism is more likely to occur when participation is anonymous.

Questions 6–10 are based on the following passage.

Passage I

Described by the psychologist B. F. Skinner, operant conditioning posits that learning can be understood by the interaction between reinforcers and stimuli. Studies from both comparative and human psychology have supported Skinner's initial findings and expanded upon them.

The following figure shows a hypothetical example of various operant conditioning trials. During these trials, when a rat pressed a bar (as indicated by the hash mark on the graph), the behavior was reinforced by the presentation of a food pellet. The reinforcement schedule differs in each cell of the figure. Time is displayed on the *x*-axis and cumulative responses (bar presses) is displayed on the *y*-axis.

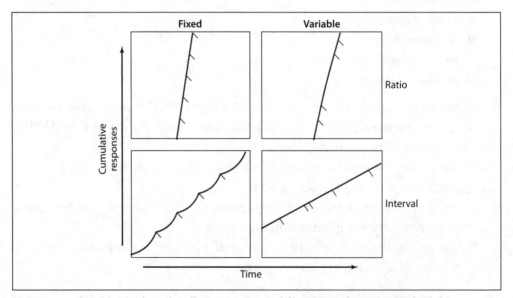

Operant conditioning with each cell representing a different reinforcement schedule.

47

SECTION 3:
Psychological,
Social, and
Biological
Foundations
of Behavior

6. Based on the figure and the concept of operant conditioning, which type of response leads to an increased cumulative response and is most likely to result in a more persistent conditioned response?
    A. fixed-ratio
    B. variable-ratio
    C. fixed-interval
    D. variable-interval

7. What would MOST likely happen if, after the bar press, reinforcement was delayed (e.g., a time lag occurred before presentation of the food pellet)?
    A. Conditioning would occur faster, and the slope in each cell of the graph would be steeper.
    B. Conditioning would occur faster but only for the variable reinforcement conditions.
    C. Conditioning would occur more slowly, and the slope in each cell of the graph would be flatter.
    D. Conditioning would occur more slowly but only for the variable reinforcement conditions.

8. Imagine that you are watching a rat complete one of the tasks in the figure above. The rat is pressing the bar at a very high rate and takes a short break from pressing the bar each time the food pellet is delivered. What type of reinforcement schedule are you MOST likely watching?
    A. variable-interval
    B. variable-ratio
    C. fixed-interval
    D. fixed-ratio

9. Based on the ratio-reinforcing graphs, for both fixed and variable conditions, which of the following would you expect?
    A. a predictable response rate for both and a lower resistance to extinction in the variable condition
    B. longer breaks between bar presses for the fixed condition and a higher resistance to extinction
    C. a predictable response rate for both and a greater resistance to extinction in the variable condition
    D. longer breaks between bar presses for the variable condition and a lower resistance to extinction.

10. Which of the following is true about conditioning?
    A. In operant conditioning the stimulus behavior always precedes the reinforcement or punishment.
    B. Operant conditioning can be used on animals while classical conditioning cannot be used.
    C. Classical conditioning can explain all learning conditions, but operant conditioning is often used for simplicity.
    D. In classical conditioning the reinforcement must never be paired with unconditioned stimulus.

Questions 11–15 are based on the following passage.

Passage II

In psychology, research examining moral development has typically focused on age-related differences. One such approach is Lawrence Kohlberg's theory that individuals progress through three levels of morality: preconventional, conventional, and postconventional. Kohlberg identified these levels based on participants' reactions to stories that present moral dilemmas. For example, participants were asked to respond to a story in which a poor man named Heinz steals a drug for his wife who would die without the drug.

The following figure depicts the moral reasoning levels that Kohlberg found within each age group on his scale. In each graph, the proportion of responders tested who showed the indicated level of moral reasoning is shown on the y-axis and the age of the responders is shown on the x-axis.

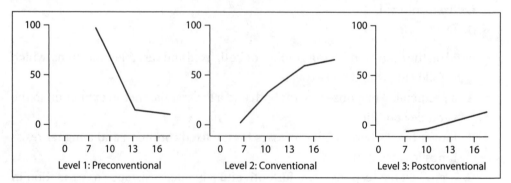

Representations of performance on Kohlberg's task with proportion of responders on the y-axis and age on the x-axis.

11. If the data pattern steadied out at 17 years old, which level would be demonstrated by the greatest proportion of responders?
    A. conventional
    B. postconventional
    C. preconventional
    D. both postconventional and preconventional equally

49

SECTION 3:
Psychological,
Social, and
Biological
Foundations
of Behavior

12. Based on the data shown, when does conventional morality develop?
    A. before age seven
    B. at age seven
    C. between the ages of 7 and 16
    D. after age 16

13. Which of the following is true about Kohlberg's theory of moral development?
    A. All adults eventually reach the postconventional stage.
    B. Moral judgments can be understood in context based on stages of moral development.
    C. The majority of children are born with the ability to tell right from wrong based on constructed moral principles.
    D. Morality is predefined with specific answers that align with societal laws.

14. According to Kohlberg's theory, which of the following is a characteristic of stage 3 morality?
    A. basing decisions only to avoid punishment or reward
    B. basing decisions on society's rules and the avoidance of punishment
    C. basing decisions on social approval of peers rather than on laws
    D. basing decisions on personally constructed moral principles rather than on societal teachings

15. James is a manager at a store. He sees a coworker temporarily abandon the check-out desk in order to help an elderly customer to her car. This act is a violation of company policy. James reports the coworker to corporate management for discipline. James is MOST likely in which stage of moral development?
    A. postconventional
    B. conventional
    C. preconventional
    D. adaptive

Questions 16–20 are based on the following passage.

Passage III

Researchers studying vision use various methods to investigate human perceptual experience. Research on spectral sensitivity of the rod receptors (scattered throughout the retina) and cone visual receptors (mainly concentrated in the fovea area of the retina) highlights the relationship between perception and physiology.

Signal detection methods have been used to measure the differences in how perception adjusts to low light environments. Participant responses can be plotted based on sensitivity versus length of time in the dark. The dark adaptation curve can be plotted showing how rods and cones differ in their sensitivity to light over time.

The following graph shows a plot of three calculated dark adaptation curves.

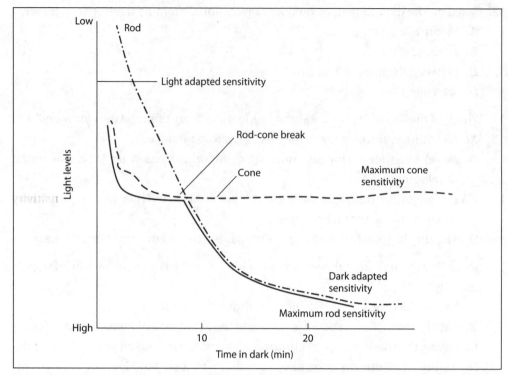

Three dark adaptation curves. Both dashed lines indicate receptor-specific curves, while the solid line is a plot of human light sensitivity with both receptor types included.

16. The dark adaptation curve can be plotted by asking participants to fixate on a specific point and then using signal detection methods with a test light. What is the MOST likely way that researchers would be able to isolate the responses of each receptor type, based on the physiology of the eye?
    A. by using colored versus white lights to differentially activate the rods and cones
    B. by changing the location of the test light from the focal point to the periphery
    C. by asking participants to cover one eye while performing the comparison tasks
    D. by alternating the brightness using flashing lights in order to preferentially activate one receptor type rather than the other

17. Signal detection methods are used to plot the dark adaptation curve. Based on these methods, what would be the threshold used for correctly detecting the presence of the test light?
    A. A participant is considered to have detected the light if he or she can identify the comparison light presence 50% of the time.
    B. A participant is considered to have detected the light if he or she can identify the comparison light presence 25% of the time.
    C. A participant is considered to have detected the light if he or she can identify the comparison light presence 75% of the time.
    D. Any time a participant identifies a light to be present, the light is considered to have been perceived.

51

SECTION 3:
Psychological,
Social, and
Biological
Foundations
of Behavior

18. Based on the dark adaptation curves, which of the following statements is true?
    A. Rods are more sensitive than cones after five minutes in the dark.
    B. Cones are more sensitive than rods after 15 minutes in the dark.
    C. Rods are more sensitive than cones at the rod-cone break.
    D. Rods are more sensitive than cones after 20 minutes in the dark.

19. Which of the following statements is true?
    A. Rods are responsible for color vision, which explains color sensitivity under low light conditions.
    B. Cones are responsible for color vision, which explains greater color sensitivity under low light conditions.
    C. Rods do not respond preferentially to wavelengths in the light spectrum, which explains why colors are not detectable in low light conditions.
    D. Both rods and cones respond to specific colors in the light spectrum; loss of color vision in dark conditions is the result of fewer photons of light.

20. What is a likely explanation for increased rod sensitivity after the rod-cone break? Select the most correct statement based on the research described above and the physiology of the eye.
    A. Cones are poorer at light adaptation because large groups of them are connected to one interneuron.
    B. Cones are better at light adaptation because they respond to specific wavelengths of light.
    C. Rods are poorer at light adaptation because they are less prone to pigment bleaching.
    D. Rods are better at light adaptation because large groups of them are connected to one interneuron.

Questions 21–25 are based on the following passage.

Passage IV

Research has examined how the presence of others affects how humans behave in different social contexts. This research has examined performance for different types of tasks and has also evaluated how group size affects performance.

   The following hypothetical data set represents the amount of time an individual devotes to solving mathematical word problems. In this example, effort is measured by the amount of time spent working to solve a multistep word problem either using algebra or calculus. The time spent by the individual was measured for each type of task when performed alone and when performed in a group. In the graph, the number of minutes spent by the individual is shown on the y-axis and the math category is shown on the x-axis.

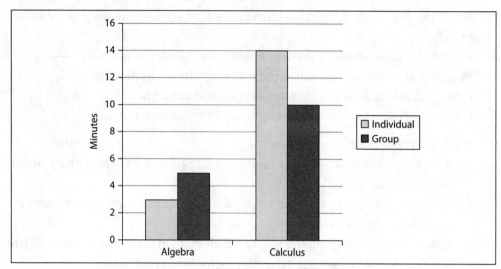

Number of minutes an individual spends to solve math problems.

21. Based on the graph, which of the following statements is true?
    A. The individual spent a longer amount of time solving calculus problems in a group compared to solving calculus problems alone.
    B. The individual spent about the same amount of time solving calculus problems in a group relative to solving them alone.
    C. The individual spent a longer amount of time solving algebra problems alone relative to solving them in a group.
    D. The individual spent a longer amount of time solving algebra problems in a group compared to solving them alone.

22. Based on research examining group performance, which of the following terms BEST explains why the individual spent less effort on solving calculus word problems when working as part of a group?
    A. social facilitation
    B. social loafing
    C. deindividuation
    D. bystander effect

23. Based on the research examining group performance, which of the following terms BEST explains why the individual spent more effort on solving algebra word problems when working as part of a group?
    A. social facilitation
    B. social loafing
    C. deindividuation
    D. bystander effect

53

SECTION 3:
Psychological,
Social, and
Biological
Foundations
of Behavior

24. What would you expect to be the MOST likely result if the complexity of the calculus problems increased (e.g., doubled in length and number of steps)?
    A. The individual would step up and expend more effort on solving the problems because he or she would feel more personally responsible.
    B. The individual would reduce the amount of effort spent on solving the problems because he or she would assume that others would step up to complete the task.
    C. The group would likely subdivide the problems into smaller tasks resulting in more individual effort overall.
    D. The amount of effort would remain unchanged.

25. Based on research examining social loafing, which of the following is true?
    A. The effort expended is the result of the participant's perception of diffusion of responsibility.
    B. The effort expended is influenced by the physical limitations that result from group work.
    C. Effort coordination explains all differences in performance for group activities.
    D. The effort expended is the result of expectations from others about an individual's work in a group.

Questions 26–30 are based on the following passage.

Passage V

Evolutionary psychology has advanced our understanding of mate selection in humans. A prominent researcher named David Buss coordinated wide-ranging research to investigate the evolutionary theory of mate selection across a wide range of cultures.

The following graphs represent female and male responses to a questionnaire about the relative importance of certain attributes of prospective mates. The first graph

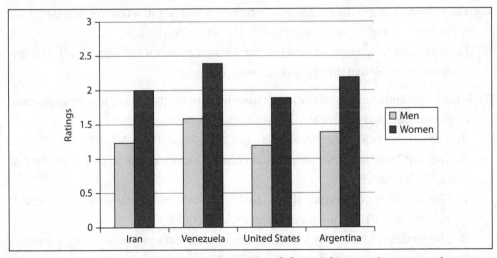

Men's and women's ratings of the importance of financial status in prospective mates. *Source*: Data from D. M. Buss. "Sex differences in human mate preferences: Evolutionary hypotheses tested in 37 cultures." *Behavioral and Brain Sciences*, 1989:12(1), 1–49.

shows how men and women in different countries rated the importance of prospective mates' financial status on a scale of 0 to 3. The second graph shows how men and women in the same four countries rated the importance of prospective mates' physical attractiveness on a scale from 0 to 3.

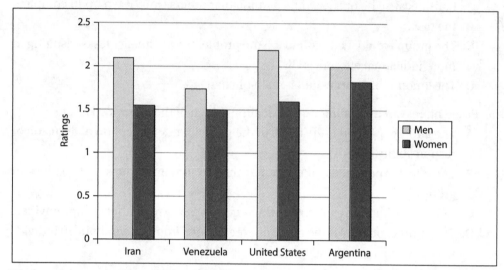

Men's and women's ratings of the importance of physical attractiveness in prospective mates. *Source*: Data from D. M. Buss. "Sex differences in human mate preferences: Evolutionary hypotheses tested in 37 cultures." *Behavioral and Brain Sciences*, 1989:12(1), 1–49.

26. Based on the graphs, which of the following statements is true?

   A. Men in the United States are the most judgmental about a partner's attractiveness in a relationship.

   B. Men and women in Venezuela rate attractiveness as equal in importance to financial status.

   C. Iran had the greatest discrepancy between men's and women's ratings on the importance of both financial status and attractiveness.

   D. Both men and women rated financial status at about the same level. The difference in relative ratings was between cultures.

27. From an evolutionary psychology perspective, what is the MOST likely explanation for the similarity in results across cultures in the data set shown?

   A. The similarity in results is a product of learned gender roles.

   B. The similarity in results shows that culture is more important than evolutionary influences.

   C. The similarity in results shows that mate selection preferences are cross-cultural and likely due to evolutionary influences.

   D. The similarity in results shows that mate selection preferences are based on experimenter expectations and gender stereotypes.

55

SECTION 3:
Psychological,
Social, and
Biological
Foundations
of Behavior

28. According to evolutionary psychology and the graphs shown, which of the following is a likely reason for the difference in how men and women rate the attributes of prospective mates?
    A. In countries where women are able to access their own financial resources, women are less likely to rate men's financial status as important because they do not need men's financial resources to raise their offspring.
    B. Women focus more on financial status than men do when selecting mates because they are driven to maximize the material resources that can be invested in children.
    C. Men are more likely to choose mates based on physical attractiveness because they have learned that is a desirable quality.
    D. In countries where plastic surgery is easily available, evolutionary psychology stops being relevant.

29. What follow-up study would be MOST likely to result in information useful to understanding mate selection from an evolutionary psychology perspective?
    A. asking participants to watch a video about stereotyping and human behavior prior to completing the survey
    B. asking participants to complete two surveys two years apart to look at how their responses have changed
    C. asking participants located in an extremely remote society to complete the same survey as used in this example study
    D. asking participants to answer only questions related to physical attractiveness

30. Which of the following is true about evolutionary psychology?
    A. Evolutionary psychology suggests that human behavior evolved due to natural selection.
    B. Evolutionary psychology focuses on cultural differences and how they influence behavior.
    C. Evolutionary psychology suggests that human behavior is more influenced by culture in more progressive societies.
    D. Evolutionary psychology suggests that human behavior is due more to learning than to natural influences.

Questions 31–35 are based on the following passage.

Passage VI

Understanding the various causes of psychological disorders is a central focus of research in psychology. Further, clinical psychologists must consider factors that influence the incidence rate and characteristics of clinical populations that they treat.

The following graphs depict data from a study by L. R. Snowden and F. K. Cheung, who examined demographic differences in the incidence rate of schizophrenia. The first figure shows the percentage rates for schizophrenia diagnosis among individuals admitted for psychiatric care who classified themselves as "African American," "White," "Hispanic American," or "Asian American and other."

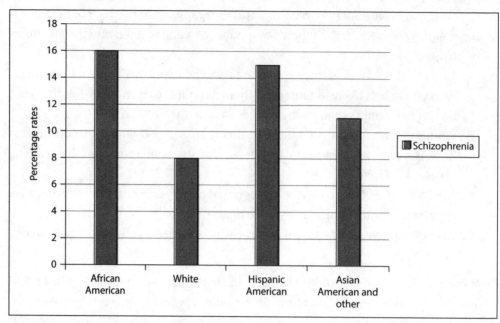

Rates of schizophrenia diagnosis for individuals admitted for psychiatric care by ethnicity.
Source: Reproduced with permission from L. R. Snowden & F. K. Cheung. "Use of inpatient mental
health services by members of ethnic minority groups." *American Psychologist*, 1990:45(3), 347.

The following graph shows the percentage rates for mood disorder diagnosis
among individuals admitted for psychiatric care, by the same ethnicity classifications.

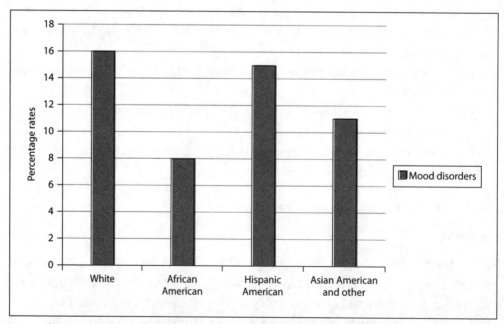

Rates of mood disorder diagnosis for individuals admitted for psychiatric care by ethnicity.
Source: Reproduced with permission from L. R. Snowden & F. K. Cheung. "Use of inpatient mental
health services by members of ethnic minority groups." *American Psychologist*, 1990:45(3), 347.

57

SECTION 3:
Psychological,
Social, and
Biological
Foundations
of Behavior

31. Based on this research, members of which ethnicity are MORE likely to be diagnosed with schizophrenia, and members of which ethnicity are MORE likely to be diagnosed with mood disorders, respectively?
    A. White; Asian American and other
    B. African American; Hispanic American
    C. African American; White
    D. Hispanic American; Hispanic American

32. Based on the data, which possible conclusion can be ruled out completely?
    A. Ethnicity has no impact on the likelihood that an individual will experience a particular mental disorder.
    B. Ethnicity is fully responsible for the likelihood an individual will experience a particular mental disorder.
    C. Clinicians see no ethnicity differences in admittance rates for some disorders.
    D. Clinicians often classify disorders based on existing biases.

33. What would be the best logical follow-up study to further examine the differences in diagnosis of mental disorders by ethnicity?
    A. Measure the social and economic status and stress of each person diagnosed with schizophrenia and mood disorder.
    B. Send the patients to a different facility to re-test the diagnosis.
    C. Compare the differences in diagnostic criteria and determine the amount of overlap between the diagnostic criteria for mood disorders and schizophrenia.
    D. Investigate why mood disorders are underrepresented in the admission samples by conducting additional surveys.

34. Based on psychological research investigating the causes of schizophrenia, which of the following is NOT true?
    A. Schizophrenia has a genetic component that can be inherited from biological parents, but genetic factors alone cannot account for the development of the disorder.
    B. The production and activity of specific chemical substances in the brain have been found to be associated with schizophrenia.
    C. Environmental factors contribute to the development of schizophrenia.
    D. A person has a 100% chance of developing schizophrenia if both of his or her parents have schizophrenia.

35. The vulnerability-stress (a.k.a. diathesis-stress) model of schizophrenia is BEST exemplified by which of the following?

   A. The more stress to which a person who is genetically predisposed to schizophrenia is exposed, the greater the likelihood that person will experience a psychotic break.

   B. Everyone becomes equally vulnerable to schizophrenia under high stress regardless of their genetic predisposition.

   C. Only negative life stressors increase the likelihood of a psychotic break in genetically predisposed individuals, while positive life stressors do not increase vulnerability.

   D. An individual is more vulnerable to schizophrenia if his or her biological family experiences stress because schizophrenia is so strongly based on genetics.

Questions 36–40 are based on the following passage.

Passage VII

Psychologists have examined how love develops over time. Their research has typically attempted to divide love into different facets whose interrelationships change over time. One such model of love developed by Robert Sternberg is shown in the following diagram and graph.

   Sternberg's model has three components: commitment, intimacy, and passion, which in combination result in multiple types of love.

Sternberg's model of love.

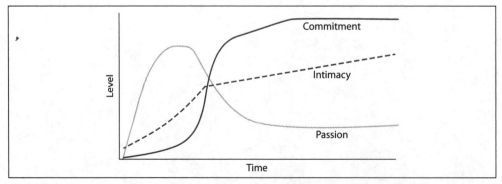

Sternberg's model of love with changes that occur over time. *Source*: From R. J. Sternberg. *The Triangle of Love: Intimacy, Passion, Commitment.* Basic Books, 1988.

59

SECTION 3:
Psychological,
Social, and
Biological
Foundations
of Behavior

36. Based on the graph, which of the following is true?
    A. Intimacy decreases over time.
    B. Passion increases rapidly early and then increases slowly over time.
    C. Commitment initially increases slowly; then it rapidly increases.
    D. Intimacy decreases as passion increases.

37. According to Sternberg's view of love, which of the following is true?
    A. Passion is unnecessary and is abandoned over time.
    B. Intimacy increases but is inherently the same as compassion.
    C. Commitment is crucial and is positively correlated to relationship stability.
    D. Passion is the most important facet for long-term love.

38. Which facet of love is characterized by intense emotion and includes tender sexual feelings?
    A. romantic love
    B. companionate love
    C. commitment
    D. intimacy

39. Which of the following statements about the types of love is MOST likely true?
    A. Fatuous love and liking can coexist in this model.
    B. Passion reaches a zenith early and then declines because you cannot like someone and be passionate about that person at the same time.
    C. In order to succeed over the long term, a relationship must maintain consummate love.
    D. Companionate love increases over time in long-term relationships.

40. Danna has been dating Mark off and on for the past two years. She enjoys the time she spends with him, but she considers him rather shallow. She still dates other people but has strong sexual feelings toward Mark. Danna is most likely experiencing which type of love?
    A. commitment
    B. companionate love
    C. intimacy
    D. infatuation

Questions 41–45 are based on the following passage.

Passage VIII

Student performance on tests has been investigated by sociologists as an indicator of how social structures influence learning. The following graph represents student performance by state on a standardized mathematics test called the Trends in International Mathematics and Science Study (TIMSS). The average TIMSS scores and standard error were calculated and are displayed in the graph. Average scores for each state are displayed individually, and the nationwide US average is also shown as a separate data point. Benchmark (target) scores are also represented in the graph.

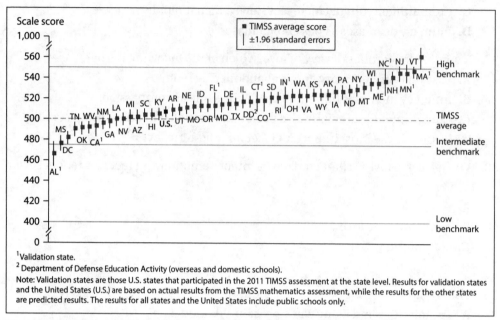

Average TIMSS score by state. *Source*: From US Department of Education, Educational Services, National Center for Education Services, National Assessment of Educational Progress (NAEP), International Association for the Evaluation of Educational Achievement (IEA), Trends in International Mathematics and Science Study (TIMSS), 2011.

41. Which of the following statements is true about the data shown in the graph?
   A. The majority of state average scores were below the national average.
   B. The majority of state average scores were above the national average.
   C. The majority of state average scores were above the high benchmark.
   D. Half of the state average scores were above the national average and half were below.

42. Using the data in the graph, a sociologist is investigating how low-scoring states are attempting to improve their performance by incorporating historically low-performing groups into local programs and services. This approach is MOST closely related to which theoretical concept?
   A. human theory
   B. functionalism
   C. symbolic interactionism
   D. conflict theory

61

SECTION 3:
Psychological,
Social, and
Biological
Foundations
of Behavior

43. Which of the following BEST indicates one way a functionalist would interpret the data in the graph?
    A. The data show that the states are equally able to reinforce the status quo in regard to their own state population.
    B. The data show the historical inequities between various state populations.
    C. The data show that education is effective in reinforcing the relative socioeconomic status (SES) status quo between various state populations.
    D. The data show that performance indicators are not relevant.

44. In terms of the overall economy, teaching in the state school system is considered to be part of which level of production?
    A. primary
    B. secondary
    C. tertiary
    D. functional

45. Jim is a sociologist who works at a public policy center in a state where TIMSS scores are well above the national average. His group is concerned with maintaining the state's lead in educational ranking in order to fend off competition from other states for high-skilled jobs. His policy center creates several initiatives to ensure that the state's schools keep their high rank and reputation for quality. Jim is MOST likely from which theoretical background?
    A. conflict theory
    B. functionalism
    C. symbolic interactionism
    D. social adaptation theory

Questions 46–50 are based on the following passage.

Passage IX

Studies collecting data on age distribution within populations have a long history in sociological research. The accompanying figure depicts the age distribution for males and females in Japan. The three graph "pyramids" show historical data for 1960 and 2010 and projections for 2060 based on current low birth rates. Each graph is separated into young, adult, and elderly populations.

Japanese population characteristics by age over time. *Source*: (for 1960 and 2010) Ministry of Internal Affairs and Communications, Population Census of Japan; (for 2060 projection) National Institute of Population and Social Security Research, Population Projections for Japan (January 2012), based on medium-variant fertility and mortality assumptions.

46. Which conclusion can be drawn from the data in the figure?
    A. The share of the elderly population in Japan will decrease over time relative to the rest of the population.
    B. The share of the young population in Japan will remain largely unchanged over time relative to the rest of the population.
    C. The share of the young population in Japan will increase over time relative to the rest of the population.
    D. The share of the elderly population in Japan will increase over time relative to the rest of the population.

47. What might be a likely result of introducing a new "transitional youth" category to data projections for the years following 2010?
    A. There would be more transitional youth in the population in 2060 than in 2020.
    B. There would be fewer transitional youth in the population in 2060 than in 2020.
    C. There would be no change in the number of transitional youth in the population in 2060 compared to 2020.
    D. There would be a decrease in the share of the elderly population in 2060 because of the addition of a new category.

48. If immigration were increased over time to compensate for the low birth rate, which of the following would MOST likely occur?
    A. Social and cultural characteristics would become more diverse across the population.
    B. Social and cultural characteristics would become more uniform across the population.
    C. Immigration would have a negligible impact because cultural groups tend not to change over time.
    D. The age distribution structure within the population would remain unchanged.

63

SECTION 3:
Psychological,
Social, and
Biological
Foundations
of Behavior

49. If current age distribution trends continue in Japan, which of the following is likely in regard to the role of the elderly in society?
    A. The elderly are likely to have less influence on public policy as their share of the population declines.
    B. The elderly are likely to have more influence on public policy as their share of the population increases.
    C. The influence of the elderly on public policy is likely to be about the same in the future as it is today.
    D. The elderly are likely to have issues adapting to new societal norms and pressures.

50. If immigration were increased over time to compensate for the low birth rate, and if the immigrants became socially and culturally integrated into the native population, which of the following would be true?
    A. The racial composition of the native population would necessarily change.
    B. The ethnicity of the overall population would change.
    C. The racial composition of the immigrant population would necessarily change.
    D. The ethnicity of the overall population would remain basically the same.

Questions 51–55 are based on the following passage.

Passage X

There are multiple reasons for racial and ethnic mental health treatment disparities in the United States. These differences have implications for mental health care. The following bar graph illustrates some of these disparities.

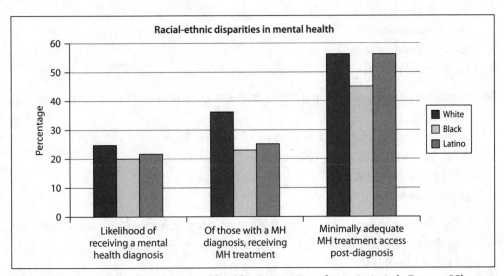

Racial and ethnic disparities in mental health. *Source*: Data from: A. A. Ault-Brutus. "Changes in racial-ethnic disparities in use and adequacy of mental health care in the United States, 1990–2003," *Psychiatric Services*, 2012:63(3), 531–540.

51. Which of the following is true based on the bar graph?
    A. Black individuals are as likely as white individuals to have access to minimally adequate mental health treatment post diagnosis.
    B. Latino individuals are as likely as white individuals to have access to minimally adequate mental health treatment post diagnosis.
    C. White individuals are as likely as Latino individuals to be diagnosed with a mental illness.
    D. White individuals are as likely as black individuals to be diagnosed with a mental illness.

52. George, an African American, was raised in surroundings of the lowest socio-economic status (SES). By working very hard in school, he earned an associate's degree in accounting. He began to take cocaine to keep up with his studies, and just before graduation began using heroin as well. He now experiences withdrawal without the drug and spends most of his time in efforts to obtain the drug. His student loans are coming due, but he has not been able to find a job because of his addiction. Based on the graph, what is the best explanation for why George is likely to continue to have an addiction problem and to remain in the lower SES?
    A. culture of poverty theory
    B. social reinforcement theory
    C. social mobility
    D. human capital

53. Lack of what form of capital is the likely primary barrier preventing George from seeking treatment and achieving social mobility?
    A. human capital
    B. financial capital
    C. environmental capital
    D. cultural capital

54. In addition to finances, what other barriers may prevent George from seeking treatment?
    A. lack of mental health providers in his geographic area
    B. stigma against seeking treatment
    C. both of the above
    D. neither of the above

55. Based on the bar graph, the individuals in which group are LEAST likely to receive treatment once they have received a mental health diagnosis?
    A. black individuals
    B. Latino individuals
    C. white individuals
    D. both Latino and black individuals

65

SECTION 3:
Psychological,
Social, and
Biological
Foundations
of Behavior

Questions 56–60 are based on the following passage.

Passage XI

High levels of sustained stress have been studied by a number of researchers. Psychological stress can create escalations in the HPA axis that shifts the body out of homeostasis.

An important theory describing the psychophysiological effects of stress was developed by the Austrian-Canadian endocrinologist Hans Selye. This theory posits a general adaptation syndrome (GAS) characterized by three stages: alarm reaction, resistance, and exhaustion.

Selye's model is shown in the following figure. The three phases are shown in order from left to right with stress plotted on the *y*-axis from low to high.

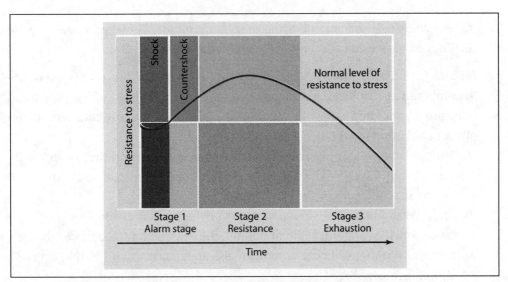

Selye's general adaptation syndrome. *Source*: Adapted from J. W. Santrock. *Adolescence*, 15th ed., McGraw-Hill Education, 2014.

56. Based on the Selye's general adaptation syndrome and your knowledge of stress physiology, which of the following is experienced during the alarm reaction stage?

   A. Bodily resources are mobilized and metabolism speeds up.
   B. Adaptability increases until it is depleted completely.
   C. Psychological resources become more moderate and sustained.
   D. People are irritable, impatient, and angry.

57. A person who is going through a divorce constantly complains about feeling tired, avoids family members who disapprove of the divorce, spends time with supportive friends, and engages in meditation in an effort to control feelings of irritation and anger. Which phase of GAS is the person MOST likely in, and how long might this condition last?

   A. Shock; the reaction will only last for a few days.
   B. Countershock; the reaction can persist for hours, days, or years.
   C. Exhaustion; the reaction will last for only a few days.
   D. Resistance; the reaction can persist for hours, days, or years.

58. Which of the following statements is true based on GAS theory?

   A. Resistance reactions are not adaptive and should be avoided.
   B. Resistance reactions are activities to reduce the impact of stress and avoid exhaustion.
   C. Physiological exhaustion is a necessary stage for any stress response.
   D. Physiological exhaustion results in increased stress.

59. An interpretation of the GAS theory posits that stressful life events occurring in combination can damage physical health. Extrapolating from the graph and integrating your knowledge of stress physiology, how would multiple simultaneous stressful events affect an individual?

   A. Multiple stressors would allow a person to repeatedly restart the process in the alarm stage, which would help that person improve resistance to stress and avoid exhaustion.
   B. Multiple simultaneous stressors may overwhelm an individual's stress resistance activities and push him or her into the exhaustion stage more quickly.
   C. It would not matter because individuals rarely encounter multiple stressors simultaneously.
   D. Stressful life events are difficult to classify or study, so we cannot begin to guess how multiple stressors would affect people.

60. Jeremy was driving on a dark road at night when a deer suddenly ran out of the brush and narrowly missed his car. Jeremy realized that there were likely more deer along the road. With his heart pounding, he turned off the road and continued to a lighted expressway with high fences. According to Selye's general adaptation syndrome theory, Jeremy was likely experiencing which of the following?

   A. a resistance reaction
   B. an alarm reaction
   C. physiological exhaustion
   D. autonomic rebound

67

SECTION 3:
Psychological,
Social, and
Biological
Foundations
of Behavior

Questions 61–65 are based on the following passage.

Passage XII

Researchers have long studied human memory. In a classic series of studies, the German psychologist Hermann Ebbinghaus investigated the storage and recall of information in memory. Based on his findings, he developed the so-called forgetting curve, a way of illustrating the rate at which people forget the information they have learned. The forgetting curve has been studied in a variety of different environments and for a variety of different stimuli.

On day 1 of a memory research study, participants were asked to learn a list of items. Researchers then tracked the proportion of the list that the participants remembered as time passed. On day 2, some participants were asked to relearn the list. Again, the proportion remembered was tracked over time. On day 3, some participants were asked to relearn the list a second time, and the proportion they remembered was tracked over time. On day 4, some participants were asked to relearn the list a third time, and the proportion they remembered was tracked over time.

The data from this study produced the following set of forgetting curves. Each line represents the memory of the learned or relearned list. The proportion of the list remembered is shown on the *y*-axis (memory), and the time interval for forgetting is shown on the *x*-axis (time remembered in days).

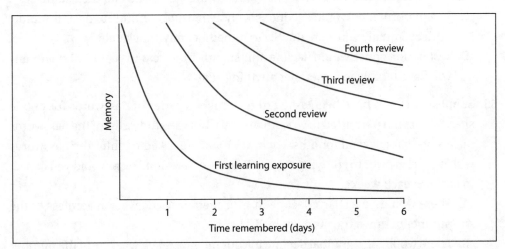

Forgetting curves. Each curve represents the memory of a learned or relearned list.

61. Based on the graph, which of the following statements BEST characterizes forgetting?
    A. Most forgetting occurs gradually over a long period of time.
    B. Most forgetting occurs after only a few days.
    C. Most forgetting occurs soon after information is learned.
    D. Most forgetting occurs at a constant rate over time.

62. The relearning periods shown in the graph indicate what about each relearning episode?

    A. Relearning has no impact on the proportion of a list remembered over time.
    B. Relearning reduces the proportion of a list remembered over time.
    C. Relearning improves memory only following the first relearning episode.
    D. Relearning increases the proportion of a list remembered over time.

63. Which of the following statements is FALSE based on the data shown in the graph?

    A. The greatest difference in retention levels occurs between learning time one and time two.
    B. Relearning is positively correlated with retention of information, but information loss still occurs over time.
    C. Relearning must occur at least four times for optimal retention.
    D. Relearning impacts the rate of forgetting only after several relearning episodes.

64. Suppose that one summer you take a training course on the maintenance and service of a certain piece of complex machinery. At the end of the course, you take a qualifying test. If you retake the test every summer for the next few years, based on the graph, how would you expect to perform on the test?

    A. Test performance would decline sharply at first but decline less and less in later years.
    B. Test performance would decline gradually over the years and then stabilize.
    C. Test performance would decline sharply at first and continue to decline rapidly until eventually you were unable to remember anything at all.
    D. Test performance would decline only slightly from year to year until eventually you were unable to remember anything at all.

65. Suppose that you have been asked to remember a series of passwords for online sites. You are not permitted to write them down but can study a list of the passwords once a week for several months. Each week you are asked to enter the passwords with no errors prior to studying the list. Based on the graph, how would you expect to perform each week?

    A. There would be a sharp decline in your memory each week regardless of the number of times you studied the list.
    B. There would be a gradual decline in your memory each week until the number of remembered passwords stabilized.
    C. There would be a gradual decline in your memory each week regardless of the number of times you studied the list.
    D. There would be a significant decline in your memory in the first week, but the decline would become less abrupt each week after you studied the list.

STOP. This is the end of Section 3.

Critical Analysis and Reasoning Skills

60 Questions   **Time Limit: 90 Minutes**

Directions: This section includes nine reading passages. Each passage is followed by a group of questions. Read each passage, and then select the one best answer to each question based on what you have read.

Questions 1–6 are based on the following passage.

Passage I

According to Professor John MacKinnon, certain places are more likely than others to house new or rediscovered species. First, scientists should look in areas that are geologically stable. Areas with regular earthquakes or volcanic eruptions are less likely to contain species that go back thousands of years because, obviously, the frequent upheavals are not conducive to steady growth or a comfortable way of life. Second, scientists are most likely to find undiscovered or rediscovered species in remote, isolated areas. Cultivated areas are inhospitable to many animals. Often, cultivation eliminates the trees or shrubs that house and protect animal life. A stable climate is a third thing to look for. Stability of climate ensures that the animals that live in the region have had no reason to leave for warmer or wetter environments.

Although most of the recent discoveries and rediscoveries of animal species have taken place in tropical, humid regions, some have occurred in rarely explored mountain habitats. A fourth key thing scientists should look for, according to MacKinnon, is an area with a variety of unusual species that are specific to that area. Of course, this requirement refers back to requirement number two, isolation. An area that is very isolated or difficult to access will naturally have species that cannot be found anywhere else.

In 1994 American biologist Peter Zahler took his second trip to the isolated valleys of the Diamer region in northern Pakistan. He was searching for the woolly flying squirrel, a dog-sized squirrel last seen in 1924. As he describes it, he had narrowed down his search to two animals, using the criteria *mammal, not too small, relatively unknown,* and *in need of conservation intervention.* Because he did not wish to spend time in the steamy environment of the Congo basin, he eliminated the aquatic genet from his list and decided to concentrate on the woolly flying squirrel, which lived in the high Himalayas where there were fewer bugs and no tropical diseases. Working with a guide, Zahler moved from valley to valley. He quizzed the local residents about the squirrel. Many recalled hearing tales about the strange animal, but all insisted it was extinct.

Zahler continued to set traps, listen to squirrel legends, and ask questions. He dodged avalanches, skirted valleys patrolled by armed warlords, and crossed mountains on narrow goat paths. Policemen told him that the squirrels indeed existed in caves above the valley, and that they excreted a substance, *salajit*, that was used as an aphrodisiac. One day, two large, machine-gun toting men entered his camp. After some small talk, one asked whether he would be willing to pay for a live squirrel. The pair claimed to be *salajit* collectors. Zahler agreed to pay top dollar, never envisioning that two hours later, he would be presented with a woolly flying squirrel in a bag. Following that surprise, Zahler located evidence of live squirrels throughout the region. The squirrel certainly obeyed all of MacKinnon's regulations. Despite frequent avalanches, the Himalayas are a geologically stable area with a harsh but stable climate and a number of rare species. Not only were the squirrels' caves remote and isolated, it was often necessary to rappel down or climb up sheer cliffs to reach them.

Each rediscovery gives scientists a vital second chance to protect and preserve our rarest, most fragile species. With scientists and students from Pakistan, Zahler began work on a program to protect the squirrel's habitat. Only the advent of war in Afghanistan forced him to abandon the area, and he remains connected to scientists in Pakistan who are continuing the effort.

1. According to the passage, all of these are true EXCEPT
    A. woolly flying squirrels excrete an unusual substance
    B. the Himalayas contain a variety of unique species
    C. animals in a drought may leave for a wetter habitat
    D. the woolly flying squirrel vanished for 70 years

2. The discussion of the aquatic genet shows primarily that
    A. some mammals are unlikely ever to be rediscovered
    B. large mammals are more easily tracked and rediscovered
    C. endangered mammals are found in many different biomes
    D. tropical diseases affect a variety of endangered species

3. Which of MacKinnon's requirements does the home of the woolly flying squirrel meet?
    I. isolation
    II. geographic stability
    III. climatic stability
    A. I only
    B. II only
    C. I and III only
    D. I, II, and III

4. The author suggests that Zahler decided to search for the woolly flying squirrel because it
   A. lived in an area that was easily accessible
   B. was neither too small nor too tropical
   C. had been spotted recently by *salajit* collectors
   D. was a legendary creature of great renown

5. According to the passage, which of these locations would be likely to house a new species?
   I. the jungles of Borneo
   II. the mountains of western Iran
   III. the edges of the eastern Sahara
   A. I only
   B. II only
   C. I and II only
   D. II and III only

6. According to the author, rediscovery gives scientists a second chance to protect and preserve rare species. Which of the following information, if true, would most WEAKEN this argument?
   A. Ornithologists hoping for a second sighting of the long-lost ivory-billed wood-pecker have triggered a stampede of cameras and news media to the fragile forests where it was recently spotted.
   B. The Audubon Society has set aside part of a forest on Oahu as a potential breeding ground for an endangered warbler once common on several of the Hawaiian islands.
   C. The northern hairy-nosed wombat lives only in one known area, a protected section of Epping Forest National Park in central Queensland, Australia.
   D. Rodent control programs on the Galapagos Islands have managed to stem a threat to endangered petrels, and now 90 percent of their nests result in a successful hatching out of eggs.

Questions 7–12 are based on the following passage.

Passage II

Beaten down, the world against them, exhausted—such was the self-assessment of the Beat Generation, as defined by Jack Kerouac in a 1948 conversation that became part of a 1952 *New York Times* article. At that time, the Beats were in their infancy. In the early '40s, Kerouac attended Columbia University on a football scholarship, but a leg injury ended his football career and forced him to drop out of school. His brief sojourn with the Merchant Marine and the Navy ended badly, and Kerouac limped back to New York to rejoin friends at Columbia, meeting student Allen Ginsberg and the older William S. Burroughs as he did so. Most of Kerouac's friends had come of age during World War II, just as Ernest Hemingway and his friends had done during World War I. Just as Hemingway's generation was "Lost," the new generation was "Beat." They found it impossible to find a place in the new, postwar economy. They lived in toxic, brutal poverty and moved constantly, and many of them struggled to find publishers for their oddly constructed, turbulent writings.

Kerouac would be the first of his friends to find a publisher, for his first novel, the rather pedestrian *The Town and the City* published in 1950. The following year, he traveled cross-country with his friend Neal Cassady, a trip that would inspire his most famous work, *On the Road*. Perhaps as much as any Beat work, this frenetic work illustrated the Beat dislike of conformity and desire for movement and new experiences.

Kerouac would continue to write prolifically in the seven years it took to get *On the Road* published. Meanwhile, Burroughs published *Junkie*, an autobiographical tome on addiction, and Ginsberg published his seminal work, the stream-of-consciousness poem "Howl." "I saw the best minds of my generation destroyed by madness . . . " cried the poet, summing up again the powerlessness of the Beat Generation. Ginsberg used street vernacular and rhythms inspired by the jazz scene of the '50s.

The Beat scene was peripatetic, moving from New York to San Francisco (where "Howl" was published) and later to the left bank in Paris, where Hemingway's Lost scene had emigrated many years earlier. Ginsberg left San Francisco for Paris when his poem "Howl" became the subject of an obscenity trial for its use of colloquial speech and its openness about drugs and homosexuality. He traveled from Paris to Tangier, where Burroughs was living, and helped Burroughs assemble the manuscript of his most famous and infamous work, *Naked Lunch*. Burroughs's book would be published in Paris in 1959 and then in the United States in 1962; again, it would be the center of a long obscenity trial. Both "Howl" and *Naked Lunch* emerged from their trials unscathed; the obscenity charges were determined to be unfounded, and the trials loosened some of the definitions that had bound American literature. In addition, of course, the publicity put the Beats on the front pages of newspapers nationwide.

The Beats were of their time, and they transcended their time. The highway system that crisscrossed the United States in the 1950s gave them the power to move. Suburbia and the man in the gray flannel suit gave them something to despise. The cold war gave them angst and disillusionment. Jazz and the drug culture gave them a way out. Without the Beats to pave the way, sixties culture would have looked quite different, and the gay liberation movement of the 1970s might never have come to pass.

7. The author compares the Beat Generation to the Lost Generation in terms of their
   A. poverty
   B. openness
   C. prolific output
   D. alienation

8. In the context of the passage, the word *culture* is used primarily to mean
   A. "nation"
   B. "sophistication"
   C. "way of life"
   D. "ethnicity"

9. The discussion of Burroughs's obscenity trial best illustrates the author's point that
   A. the Beat scene was peripatetic
   B. the Beats affected definitions of literature
   C. the Beats were inspired by jazz and angst
   D. the Beats transcended their time

10. Which of the following assertions does the author support with an example?
    I. Kerouac continued to write prior to the publication of *On the Road*.
    II. The drug culture affected the lives and writings of some Beats.
    III. Sixties culture was influenced by the work of the Beats.
    A. I only
    B. II only
    C. I and III only
    D. II and III only

11. Gregory Corso, another important figure in the Beat crowd, once wrote a poem in the shape of a mushroom cloud entitled "Bomb." If the author included this information in the passage, it would probably be used to
    A. contrast with Ginsberg's description of "the best minds of my generation"
    B. represent an example of colloquial speech in Beat poetry and prose
    C. support the notion that the cold war colored the Beats' work with angst
    D. illustrate the Beats' dislike for conformity and the postwar economy

12. Suppose the Beat writers were omitted from a major anthology of American literature. This would challenge the author's assertion that
    A. the Beats affected the gay liberation movement
    B. the Beats' writing was turbulent and difficult
    C. the Beats often struggled to find publishers
    D. the Beats transcended their time

Questions 13–18 are based on the following passage.

Passage III

Aluminum is the most abundant metallic element in the Earth's crust, but it is never found naturally as an element. Instead, it always appears naturally in its oxidized form as a hydroxide we call bauxite.

Bauxite occurs in three main forms. The forms vary in the number of molecules of water it takes for hydration and in the crystalline structure of the molecule. Gibbsite is a trihydrate form [$Al(OH)_3$]. Bohmite and diaspore are monohydrates [$AlO(OH)$]. Of the three, the main form that is mined is gibbsite. Bauxite may be hard or soft, and it comes in a variety of colors that range from white to red.

Bauxite is formed due to the weathering of alumina-bearing rocks. It often appears as an extensive blanket of ore and is usually mined using surface mining techniques. By far the largest consumers of aluminum are the United States, Japan, and Germany, but except for a little in Texas and Arkansas, bauxite is nearly nonexistent there. The major producers of bauxite are Australia, which produces around 40 percent of the world's supply, and Guinea, in West Africa. The United States gets much of its supply from Brazil and Jamaica.

The extraction of aluminum from bauxite requires three stages. First, the ore is mined. Then it is refined to recover alumina. Finally, the alumina is smelted to produce aluminum.

The mining is done via the open-cut method. Bulldozers remove the topsoil, and excavators or other types of power machinery are used to remove the underlying layer of bauxite. The bauxite may be washed to remove clay and other detritus.

Refining is done via the Bayer refining process, named after its inventor, Karl Bayer. Ground bauxite is fed into a digester, where it is mixed with a caustic soda. The aluminum oxide reacts with the soda to form a solution of sodium aluminate and a precipitate of sodium aluminium silicate. The solution is separated from the silicate through washing and pumping, and the alumina is precipitated from the solution, where it appears as crystals of alumina hydrate. The crystals are washed again to remove any remaining solution. Then they are heated to remove water, leaving the gritty alumina.

Smelting is done via the Hall-Heroult smelting process. An electric current is passed through a molten solution of alumina and cryolite, which is in a cell lined at the bottom and top with carbon. This forces the oxygen to combine with the carbon at the top of the cell, making carbon dioxide, while the molten metallic aluminum collects at the bottom of the cell, where it is siphoned off, cleaned up, and cast into bars, sheets, or whatever form is needed.

As with all mining of metals, bauxite mining presents certain hazards. Along with the usual mining issues of degraded soil and polluted runoff, chief among them is the omnipresent bauxite dust, which clogs machinery and lungs, sometimes for miles around the mining site. Jamaica and Brazil have seen widespread protests recently against the major bauxite mining companies, which continue to insist that no link between bauxite dust and pervasive lung problems has been proved.

13. In the context of the passage, the word *refined* means
    A. "superior"
    B. "polished"
    C. "processed"
    D. "restricted"

14. The discussion of protests shows primarily that
    A. bauxite mining takes place in the Third World
    B. workers are starting to fight back against the dangers of mining
    C. mining companies have misled people for decades
    D. the government of Brazil works with the mining companies

15. The passage suggests that the author would MOST likely believe that
    A. bauxite mining poses health problems
    B. the United States should use less aluminum
    C. Australian bauxite is the best quality
    D. Karl Bayer was something of a genius

16. All of these are produced by the Bayer process EXCEPT
    A. sodium aluminum silicate
    B. sodium aluminate
    C. aluminum manganese
    D. alumina hydrate

17. According to the passage, the most commonly mined form of bauxite contains
    A. carbon dioxide
    B. iron by-products
    C. caustic soda
    D. three molecules of water

18. The process by which aluminum is extracted from bauxite is most similar to
    A. the building of steel bridges
    B. the making of copper tubing
    C. the manufacturing of glass
    D. the mixing of cement

Questions 19–25 are based on the following passage.

Passage IV

"I acknowledge Shakespeare to be the world's greatest dramatic poet, but regret that no parent could place the uncorrected book in the hands of his daughter, and therefore I have prepared the Family Shakespeare."

Thus did Thomas Bowdler, a self-appointed editor trained as a physician, explain his creation of a children's edition of Shakespeare that omitted some characters completely, toned down language he considered objectionable, and euphemized such shocking situations as Ophelia's suicide—an accident in Bowdler's version.

Bowdler was hardly the first to tone down the Bard. Poet laureate Nahum Tate rewrote *King Lear*, banishing the Fool entirely and giving the play a happy ending. His version was staged regularly from the 1680s through the eighteenth century.

Thomas Bowdler was, from all the evidence, a less likely editor. He was born in 1754 near Bath, England, to a wealthy family. He studied medicine but never really practiced, preferring to exercise philanthropy and to play chess, at which he was a master. In his retirement, he decided to try his hand at editorial work. Shakespeare's dramas were his first project. He added nothing to the texts, but by cutting and paraphrasing strove to remove anything that "could give just offense to the religious and virtuous mind."

The result was a 10-volume expurgated version that was criticized widely, although hardly universally. The famed British poet Algernon Swinburne remarked that "no man ever did better service to Shakespeare than the man who made it possible to put him into the hands of intelligent and imaginative children."

There is some indication that Bowdler's sister Harriet did the actual editing of Shakespeare's text. She was a poet and editor in her own right, and clearly more qualified than her brother to lay hands on the Bard of Avon. She may have published the expurgated edition anonymously before allowing her brother to take over the rights. If this is so, it is unsurprising that Harriet would not have wanted her name on the book. If the original Shakespeare were truly objectionable, then it would have been doubly so for a well-bred, unmarried Englishwoman of the day.

Bowdler went on to create children's versions of the Old Testament and of Edward Gibbons's *History of the Decline and Fall of the Roman Empire*, although neither achieved either the success or ridicule of his Shakespeare. Today, of course, we know Bowdler not for his good works, but instead for the eponym derived from his good name. To *bowdlerize* is to censor or amend a written work, often with a connotation of prudishness. The process for which Bowdler is known is one that continues to the present day, as texts deemed too difficult for today's high schoolers are "dumbed-down," library editions of *The Adventures of Huckleberry Finn* have the "n-word" blacked out, and middle-school productions of popular Broadway plays have all expletives deleted. We would be hard-pressed to say that we live in a prudish era, but some of the same impulses that drove Thomas and Harriet Bowdler still exist today.

19. The main argument of the final paragraph is that
    A. Bowdler did a disservice to the readers of his works
    B. Bowdler's edited texts have long since vanished into history
    C. we continue to bowdlerize texts to the present day
    D. today we look at Bowdler as a negative influence on writing

20. The passage implies that Bowdler's sister was a more likely editor than he because
    A. she would have been truly offended by Shakespeare's plots
    B. unlike her brother, she was a published writer and editor
    C. Bowdler was known for his misuse of the English language
    D. women of the time were more likely to read Shakespeare

21. The passage suggests that Bowdler was influenced by
    A. prudery
    B. erudition
    C. a poet laureate
    D. a dream

22. The mention of Nahum Tate shows primarily that
    A. few dared to change Shakespeare's works during his lifetime
    B. actors and directors often changed Shakespeare's words to suit their talents
    C. different versions of *King Lear* were used depending on the audience
    D. the Bowdlers were not the first to alter Shakespeare's texts

23. Based on the information in this passage, which of these would NOT be bowdlerization?
    I. translating a Japanese folktale into English
    II. eliminating references to witches from a fairy tale
    III. burning copies of *The Satanic Verses*
    A. I only
    B. II only
    C. I and III only
    D. II and III only

24. The author's claim that Bowdler's Shakespeare was not unanimously criticized is supported by
    A. a quotation from Algernon Swinburne
    B. reference to later children's works by Bowdler
    C. the definition of the eponym formed from his name
    D. the example of Ophelia's revised "suicide"

25. Given the information in the passage, if a bowdlerized version of Shakespeare were available to parents today, which of the following outcomes would MOST likely occur?
    A. Some would ridicule it, and others would buy it.
    B. No one would take it or its author seriously.
    C. Most students would find it too difficult to read.
    D. It would be a dismal failure and be taken off the market.

Questions 26–33 are based on the following passage.

Passage V

The Nobel Peace Prize has often engendered controversy. The Red Cross, yes, but Henry Kissinger? Mother Teresa, perhaps, but Yasser Arafat? Surprisingly, a loud and ongoing controversy surrounds a choice that at first look seems most benign—that of the Guatemalan freedom fighter, Rigoberta Menchú Tum.

Rigoberta Menchú was born in 1959 to a poor Mayan family in Guatemala. At the time of her birth, General Ydígoras Fuentes had just seized power, following the assassination of Colonel Castillo Armas. The year she turned one, there was a failed coup by a military group, many of whom fled to the countryside and would return to lead the rebellion that would wax and wane for the next 36 years.

Guatemala was divided into factions for that entire period, as military governments controlled the nation and guerilla groups controlled the countryside. At the same time, right-wing vigilantes led a campaign of torture and assassination, eliminating students and peasants they deemed to be allied with the guerillas.

In the countryside where Rigoberta lived, the battles were largely over control of farmland. Rigoberta's father was taken into custody and tortured when the army believed he had assisted in the assassination of a plantation owner. Following a rout of the guerillas by the army, the guerillas regrouped and began to take their fight to the capital, beginning a long series of assassinations of government figures.

Rigoberta, her father, and some of her siblings joined the Committee of the Peasant Union (CUC). In rapid succession, Rigoberta lost her brother, father, and mother to the army's own assassination squads. Rigoberta, though only in her early 20s, became a key figure in the resistance, traveling from village to village to educate the Mayan peasants in overcoming oppression, and leading demonstrations in Guatemala City.

Soon Rigoberta was herself a target. She fled to Mexico and continued her life as an organizer, concentrating her focus on peasants' rights. She participated in the founding of the United Representation of the Guatemalan Opposition (RUOG). This period was the most violent of the entire Guatemalan civil war. Under the new president, General Efrain Ríos Montt, massacres of civilians became an everyday occurrence.

Rigoberta traveled to Paris, where she sat down and dictated her life story to anthropologist Elisabeth Burgos Debray. This story, titled *I, Rigoberta Menchú, an Indian Woman in Guatemala*, would galvanize world attention to the plight of Guatemala. Shortly thereafter, Ríos Montt was overthrown in a coup, and the slow work of democratizing Guatemala began. In 1992, Rigoberta would win the Nobel Peace Prize for her life and work.

The controversy is all about the book. It began when anthropologist David Stoll began independent research on the same era about which Rigoberta dictated and discovered discrepancies in her recall of events. Massacres she described were not remembered by the locals; one of her brothers died by shooting rather than by fire, dates were incorrect, and so on. Stoll's discoveries were enough to roil up conservative historians and columnists, who declared Rigoberta's book the grossest propaganda and her career, therefore, unworthy of the Nobel Prize. Not surprisingly, this brought forth charges of racism, sexism, and cultural ignorance from the other side.

The Nobel Committee maintained a stiff upper lip throughout the political back-and-forth and still insists that Rigoberta's prize had to do with her documented good works and not with her personal recorded history. Rigoberta's book is still widely taught, and her place in the history of Central American peasant revolutions seems assured.

26. Which choice(s) by the Nobel Committee does the author seem to indicate was undeserved?
    I. Rigoberta Menchú
    II. Henry Kissinger
    III. The Red Cross
    A. I only
    B. II only
    C. I and III only
    D. II and III only

27. In the context of the passage, the word *custody* means
    A. "fortification"
    B. "safekeeping"
    C. "incarceration"
    D. "supervision"

28. Which of the following statements is/are NOT presented as evidence that Rigoberta may have falsified her autobiography?
    I. Massacres she described were not remembered by the locals.
    II. One of her brothers died by shooting rather than by fire.
    III. Rigoberta dictated her life story to anthropologist Debray.
    A. I only
    B. I and II only
    C. III only
    D. II and III only

29. According to the passage, why did Rigoberta leave Guatemala?
    A. She wanted to alert the world to the problems of the peasants.
    B. She was under fire from the army's assassination squads.
    C. She was invited to Paris to dictate her personal memoirs.
    D. She no longer cared to stay after her family was murdered.

30. The author's claim that Rigoberta's book is still widely taught could BEST be supported by the inclusion of
    A. two students' comments on the ongoing controversy
    B. data on the sales for her book from publication until the present day
    C. a record of bookstores that continue to carry her autobiography
    D. a list of universities that include her book in their required reading lists

31. Which new information, if true, would BEST support conservatives' claims that Rigoberta was a fraud?
    A. the discovery that Rigoberta was really born in early 1960
    B. findings that show Rigoberta educated thousands of Mayan peasants
    C. the discovery that neither Rigoberta nor her parents were part of CUC
    D. findings that show Ríos Montt was overthrown by a peasant army

32. If David Stoll is to be believed, Rigoberta's autobiography seems to be an example of
    A. "truthiness," the quality of preferring facts one wishes were true to those that are true
    B. "epic," a narrative unified by a legendary hero who reflects the aspirations of a nation or race
    C. "folktale," a story of cumulative authorship from the oral tradition
    D. "manifesto," a credo or position paper in which the leader of a political movement sets forth tenets and beliefs

33. The author of the passage would probably support
    A. an inquiry that led to the removal of Rigoberta's Nobel Prize
    B. the removal of Rigoberta's autobiography from college curricula
    C. keeping Rigoberta's name in the history books as a freedom fighter
    D. granting the Nobel Prize exclusively to groups, not individuals

Questions 34–40 are based on the following passage.

Passage VI

If our knowledge of the world occurs through the weaving of narratives, as postmodernists would have us believe, then we must judge the truth of each narrative by comparing it with what we value and what we already accept as true. Any metanarrative, or overarching "big story," must be rejected because it attempts to explain away too many individual narratives.

The traditional metanarrative of American history, for example, might posit that the country was forged and tamed by white men who arrived by ship from a continent (Europe) that did not allow them the freedoms they desired. Viewing all of American history through that metanarrative, postmodernists would argue, does not allow us to consider the contributions of other groups to the country we live in today. So constructing a metanarrative can often be exclusionary.

Of course, constructing a series of smaller narratives is just as exclusionary because it frames experience in a limited way. It is easy to see this occurring if you look at any university course list today. How is it possible for American History 4111, "Imperialism and Amerindians, 1600–1840" to coexist alongside American History 4546, "American Military History and Policy"? Does English 340X, "Survey of Women's Literature," subsume or incorporate elements of English 342X, "American Indian Women Writers"? Perhaps we should pity the undergraduate student today. Lacking any overarching metanarrative to provide perspective, how can the poor student wade through the often-contradictory mininarratives being thrown his or her way?

There is no question that the old way was wrongheaded and elitist. Survey courses that emphasized the white male perspective were removed from the curriculum in the 1970s, '80s, and '90s, and for good reason. But replacing them with a smorgasbord of mininarratives risks eliminating any sense of a big picture. Can students connect the dots to define a coherent reality, or must their reality be a series of frames with no links among them?

Revising the canon was about ridding our perspective of those racist, sexist, or classist notions that insisted on a single Truth with a capital T. Of course there is no overriding Truth that applies to everyone. For everyone who believes that Thomas Jefferson was a brilliant reformer, there is someone who thinks he was a two-faced slaveholder. Yet, where does it leave us if everyone we know is approaching history, science, literature, or what have you from a slightly different angle? It's bad enough when partisan politics divides us into red states and blue states. How much worse is it to imagine ourselves clad in thousands upon thousands of shades of purple?

The clearest sign that we are not ready to abandon our metanarratives comes in the current and ongoing clash between those who accept evolutionary theory and those who accept the Bible as the written word of God. The latter grant the Earth 6000 years of life, the former give it several million more, and never the twain shall meet. Each of these viewpoints is a metanarrative, a big story that governs people's understanding of the world. Like many metanarratives, each of these completely negates the other.

So on the one hand, metanarratives don't work well because they are too exclusionary. And on the other hand, mininarratives don't work well because they are too narrow. It will be fascinating to watch the canon evolve over the next few decades and to see whether this dichotomy can ever be resolved.

34. The main argument of the passage is that
    A. metanarratives provide the best way to view the world
    B. metanarratives are usually more restrictive than mininarratives
    C. mininarratives are racist, sexist, and classist
    D. neither metanarratives nor mininarratives offer a flawless perspective

35. The passage suggests that the author would MOST likely believe that
    A. colleges should offer more courses in American history
    B. revising the canon in the late twentieth century was a bad idea
    C. students today need a more global perspective than their coursework provides
    D. divisiveness in politics is preferable to conformity or unilateralism

36. Which of the following assertions does the author support with an example?
    I. Constructing mininarratives frames experience in a limited way.
    II. We are not ready to abandon our metanarratives.
    III. Constructing a metanarrative may be exclusionary.
    A. I only
    B. III only
    C. I and II only
    D. I, II, and III

37. The ideas in this passage would be MOST useful to
    A. authors of novels in the postmodern tradition
    B. committees responsible for establishing college curricula
    C. students of ancient Roman or Greek philosophy
    D. journalists, detectives, and other seekers of truth

38. The author states that metanarratives have been replaced on campuses by a "smorgasbord" of mininarratives. The word *smorgasbord* is used to indicate
    A. freshness
    B. choice
    C. flavor
    D. foreignness

39. Based on the information in the passage, which of these might be considered a metanarrative?
    I. Marxism
    II. rationalism
    III. libertarianism
    A. I only
    B. II only
    C. II and III only
    D. I, II, and III

40. A comparison of a mininarrative to a metanarrative would be MOST similar to a comparison of
    A. a cropped photograph to a wide-angle photograph
    B. a globe to a world map
    C. a ranch-style house to a palace
    D. a single domestic turkey to a flock of wild turkeys

Questions 41–46 are based on the following passage.

Passage VII

What began as an online personal diary of sorts about a decade ago has become a multimillion-dollar-a-year business that is reshaping the nature of the media, publishing, and marketing. It has the power to catapult unknowns into celebrities, affect political careers, and even influence language. They were known first as "web logs," which evolved into "weblogs" and finally "blogs." In 2004, Merriam-Webster declared *blog* its Word of the Year.

It is estimated that more than 50 million people are blogging, and every second two new blogs are created. Most bloggers use the tool for its original purpose: periodically posting their thoughts on subjects of their choosing for others to read and comment on. But what sounds on the surface to be merely a public display of ideas is in effect changing the nature of media. Print newspapers and magazines have a staff of writers, researchers, and editors who find what they deem to be appropriate (often defined as "nonoffense") material, shape it, and present it to an audience of passive consumers. When those passive consumers use simple websites to disseminate facts and ideas of their choosing, they evolve from passive consumers to active participants, effectively blurring the line between the media and its audience.

Many bloggers choose to focus on news stories that receive little attention from traditional media outlets. They research, report, and comment on information that the public might otherwise not have easy access to. Traditional media companies have stockholders to answer to, and sometimes edit content to eliminate or reduce possible controversial material. Blogs, in comparison, thrive on controversy. Indeed, that is where they most often make their mark. Talking Points Memo, which debuted in 2000, is a left-wing political site whose staff has grown to include eight employees, including five research interns. In December 2002, the blog focused on Senator Trent Lott's comments at a political function that many deemed bigoted, a story that was virtually ignored by print, radio, and television media sources. In less than two weeks, the public outcry grew, and Lott resigned from his post as Senate majority leader.

In addition to their influence, popular bloggers are able to turn their sleuthing and private rants into dollars. Marketers looking for new and more effective ways to reach consumers are increasingly spending money on online advertising. By 2005, it was estimated that $100 million dollars' worth of blogs ads were sold. One blogger in Kentucky uses his site, fark.com, to spread his brand of humor and is earning millions of dollars in ad revenue this year, thanks to the support of theme parks, shampoos, and nutrition bars. But this is predicted to be just the tip of the blog profitability iceberg. Overall web advertising is expected to grow by 50 percent to $23.6 billion in 2010; much of that will make its way on to blogs.

41. The central thesis of the passage is that
    A. blogging was once a solitary activity, but popular blogs now have readerships in the millions
    B. advertisers are spending more money on blogs and less on traditional print and broadcasting outlets
    C. blogs are not only becoming profitable, but they are also influencing the media and the business of publishing and advertising
    D. some bloggers have become millionaires as their popular websites are replete with advertising

42. The passage implies that bloggers who want to receive, or increase current levels of, advertising revenue must
    A. strive to be more controversial
    B. build their readership
    C. include more content concerning celebrities and politicians
    D. appeal directly to marketers

43. Suppose evidence was presented to show that traditional media sources were becoming successful in their attempts to compete for blogs' advertising revenue. This new information would MOST challenge the implication that
    A. advertisers are spending money on blogs because they present a more effective way to reach consumers
    B. people choose to read blogs because they don't have to appeal to stockholders
    C. popular blogs are better at disseminating information than traditional media sources
    D. active participants blur the line between the media and its audience

44. Which of the following assertions does the author support with an example?
    I. Blogs influence language.
    II. Blogs are used by politicians to shape public discourse.
    III. Blogs disseminate information that traditional media sources neglect.
    A. I only
    B. II only
    C. I and III only
    D. I, II, and III

45. According to the passage, what is one way in which blogs are changing the nature of media?

    A. They are siphoning advertising revenue from traditional news sources.

    B. They are able to affect political careers.

    C. They allow consumers to become active participants in the dissemination of ideas.

    D. They are a public display of ideas.

46. The passage suggests that Talking Points Memo's coverage of a senator's inappropriate comments was

    A. helpful in attracting advertisers, and therefore revenue-producing

    B. designed to increase readership

    C. an ineffective way to end the senator's career

    D. at odds with news coverage provided by traditional media sources

Questions 47–53 are based on the following passage.

Passage VIII

It is perhaps too easy to think of mathematical truths as objective entities existing in the universe, simply waiting to be "discovered" by brilliant minds such as Pythagoras, Newton, and Descartes. Indeed, such a mentality may be cemented in Western minds raised in the Platonic tradition of a world of ideals that exists outside of the material world we reside in.

But new research in the fields of cognitive science and developmental psychology may be challenging this long-held belief in mathematics as a truth outside of human experience, and recasting mathematics as a product of the brain, an entity that is not discovered by man but rather created by him.

Such a radical paradigm shift has predictably met with stiff resistance, but the evidence in favor of a created mathematics rather than a discovered mathematics is compelling. Study after study has shown that all people possess an innate arithmetic. Babies as young as three or four days old can differentiate between groups of two and three items. And by the age of four months or so, an infant can see that one plus one is two and two minus one is one. Researchers discovered this startling fact by means of a simple experiment, following what is known as the violation of expectation model in developmental psychology. An infant was presented with a scenario in which a researcher held a puppet before the baby's eyes. Then a screen was moved in front of the puppet and another researcher placed a second puppet behind it. The screen was removed and if there were two puppets now visible, the infant registered no surprise (as measured by both the direction of the child's gaze and the duration of her stare). But if the screen was removed and only one puppet appeared, the infant registered perplexity at the situation.

This experiment and others like it strongly suggest that all individuals are born with certain mathematical concepts hardwired into their brains. The ability to quickly and accurately count a small number of items, called *subitizing* by psychologists, is also found in animals. Researchers using experiments similar to the violation of expectation setup described previously have found an innate mathematical ability not just in primates, our closest evolutionary cousins, but in raccoons, rats, parrots, and pigeons. These findings are consistent with the belief that mathematical thinking is a function of the structures in the brain and not a product of the outside world.

Anomalous cases involving brain injuries and disorders also support the idea that mathematical thinking arises from the organization of the brain. There is a documented case of a subject with a PhD in chemistry who suffers from acalculia, the inability to perform basic arithmetic functions. Strangely, this patient is unable to perform simple calculations such as five plus three or eight minus two, but has no problem manipulating abstract algebraic operations. This curious fact has led psychologists to conclude that the part of the brain that handles abstract algebraic operations must be different from the part of the brain that works with more concrete arithmetic functions.

47. The author probably mentions the "Platonic tradition" in order to
    A. explain why some people may be less accepting of certain conclusions
    B. demonstrate the philosophical and historical underpinnings of mathematical studies
    C. highlight another influential Western figure in mathematical thought
    D. argue that followers of non-Western philosophical traditions are more likely to agree with the author's thesis

48. The author supports the passage's main thesis with all of the following types of evidence EXCEPT
    A. experiments
    B. case studies
    C. testimonials
    D. comparisons

49. The passage implies that
    A. structures for arithmetic calculations are hardwired into the brain, but those for algebraic manipulations are not
    B. most animals are able to perform simple arithmetic operations
    C. infants at the age of three or four days can already perform simple calculations
    D. mathematical concepts are arbitrary

50. In the context of the passage, the word *curious* means
    A. "marvelous"
    B. "exotic"
    C. "odd"
    D. "novel"

51. In the discussion of the violation of expectation experiment, the author assumes that
   A. certain observable behaviors accurately indicate inner mental states
   B. the infants in the study did not know what happened to the puppets behind the screen
   C. researchers used the same types of puppets in all of the experiments
   D. animals and infants performed at similar levels of competency in the experiments

52. The central thesis of the passage is that
   A. Western philosophers were mistaken in their belief in mathematics as an objective truth
   B. research in cognitive science and developmental psychology indicates that some animals may have the same mathematical abilities as humans do
   C. a longstanding attitude toward mathematics may need to be reexamined in light of new evidence
   D. people create their own mathematical systems based on the structures in their brains

53. Suppose a team of anthropologists discovered an isolated community of individuals who possessed absolutely no mathematical ability whatsoever. This discovery would have what effect on the author's argument?
   A. It would refute it.
   B. It would support it.
   C. It would neither support nor refute it.
   D. It would be necessary to determine the cause of the individuals' lack of mathematical ability in order to say what effect it would have on the argument.

Questions 54–60 are based on the following passage.

Passage IX

Language consists of three main parts. The first is simply vocabulary, the lexicon of words available to the speaker to describe particular concepts, actions, and states. The second part is morphology, the set of rules that dictates how words and parts of words may be combined to form other words. The final part of language is syntax, the rules that combine words into phrases and sentences. It is morphology that we shall turn our attention to first.

Morphology has two major subdivisions. They are derivation and inflection. Derivation refers to those rules by which new words may be formed out of preexisting words. Inflection, sometimes commonly referred to as conjugation and declension, states how words are changed to indicate their function within a sentence.

Although common mythology holds that English is one of the most difficult languages to learn, many linguists would beg to differ. In fact, when it comes to inflection English is almost juvenile in its simplicity when compared to other languages. For example, Spanish verbs have about 50 forms, unique combinations that indicate the first, second, and third person; whether a verb is singular or plural; whether the verb is in the past, present, or future tense; and any number of moods, including the indicative, the conditional, the subjunctive, the imperative, and others. Languages from outside the Indo-European family tree may be even more complex. The Bantu language of Kivunjo has roughly half a million combinations of prefixes and suffixes for a verb. English, however, has a mere four combinations. A verb such as *to walk* is limited to the following forms: *walk, walks, walked,* and *walking.*

Although there are only four basic verb forms, the English language does have more than 13 possible inflections. It just makes do with these four forms for the various functions. English also differs significantly from many other Indo-European languages in that in English, the stem of the word can be pronounced and is in fact part of the language. In Spanish, the stem of the verb *to walk* is *camin-,* but this is not a word in the language. In order to pronounce this word, it must be conjugated and combined with a suffix. English uses the stem form of the verb for four inflections: the present tense (except for the third-person singular), the infinitive, the imperative, and the subjunctive. The verb form ending in –*s* is used in only one case, the third-person singular.

The two possible verb suffixes, –*ing* and –*ed,* are put to use in a variety of ways as well. The –*ing* ending appears in the progressive participle, the present participle, the gerund form, and the verbal adjective form. That leaves the –*ed* form to handle the remaining inflections, including the past tense, the perfect participle, the passive participle, and some verbal adjectives.

Why are there so many different inflections for verb forms that basically sound the same? Simply put, the meanings implied by the various moods are different, even if the words used are fairly similar. Compare the meaning conveyed by the simple past tense (*he walked*) to the meaning inherent in the perfect participle (*he has walked*).

54. The central thesis of the passage is that
    A. English is easier to learn than many other languages
    B. each language is unique in its major forms
    C. the English language uses a minimum of verb forms in its inflections
    D. the English language is not as rich in meaning as other languages

55. The passage suggests that the author MOST likely believes that
    A. the English language does not suffer from its lack of inflections
    B. English is the only language in which the verb stem is a word
    C. English is not as hard to learn as many think
    D. at one time the English language had more inflections

56. Which of the following assertions does the author support with an example?
    I. The English language is relatively simple in its inflections.
    II. The English language is not as hard to learn as some believe.
    III. Inflections in the English language can convey a variety of meanings.
    A. I only
    B. III only
    C. I and III only
    D. II and III only

57. The ideas presented in this passage would probably be MOST interesting to
    A. linguists
    B. language teachers
    C. psychologists
    D. translators

58. The passage indicates that a native Spanish speaker may be puzzled by the verb *to see* in which of the following sentences?
    A. I saw the car.
    B. They want to see the car.
    C. She sees the car.
    D. Seeing is believing.

59. According to the passage, which English inflection can be expressed by two different verb suffixes?
    I. the present tense
    II. the verbal adjective
    III. the present participle
    A. I only
    B. I and II only
    C. III only
    D. I, II, and III

60. The Russian language is similar to the Spanish language in that the verbs have stem forms that are not words unto themselves. From this fact, a linguist might infer that
    A. Russian verbs have roughly 50 forms
    B. the Russian language may be of the Indo-European family
    C. Russian is harder to learn than Spanish
    D. the Russian language has more inflections than the English language

STOP. This is the end of Section 4.

ANSWERS AND EXPLANATIONS

Section 1. Biological and Biochemical Foundations of Living Systems

1. **The correct answer is B.** The passage explains that in acute cases of leukemia, immature leukocytes are involved. This implies that these immature cells are abnormal and may not proliferate into normal mature leukocytes. The passage also indicates that in chronic cases of leukemia, mature leukocytes are affected so that it is possible that some unaffected immature cells may proliferate into functional mature cells. If there are some functional leukocytes, the person would be likely to survive longer without treatment.

2. **The correct answer is A.** The blood-brain barrier is a change in the permeability of blood vessels leading to the brain. Depending on the chemical composition, some drugs can cross and some cannot. Of the choices listed, it seems that if the drugs cannot reach the brain, then they have not crossed the blood-brain barrier. While choice D might seem plausible if a drug was ingested, it would not make sense for a drug that was injected.

3. **The correct answer is C.** Of the items listed in the question, the thing they all have in common is that they are mutagens or involve some genetic change. These mutations to the DNA can lead to the production of altered proteins that can be associated with cancer. While some cancers are associated with changes in cellular growth factors, this would not be the case for all cancers. The translation of proteins is directly from the mRNA, which is derived from the DNA in transcription. There would have to be a change in the DNA for the translation of proteins to be affected.

4. **The correct answer is C.** This question is simply asking about the function of antibiotics. Since a person with leukemia has abnormal leukocytes, there can be problems with the functioning of the immune system such that it does not fight infection well. Antibiotics kill bacteria cells, not viruses, and could help prevent bacterial infections in the leukemia patient who has a compromised immune system.

5. **The correct answer is A.** Some of the choices listed here relate to processes that are not unique to the cell cycle, which regulates cell division. Since cancer involves abnormal cell division, there is a problem with cell-cycle regulation. For example, protein synthesis is not a cell-cycle specific process. Purine analogs can be incorporated during DNA and RNA synthesis, which is also not cell-cycle specific. Alkylating agents interfere with DNA functioning, which is also not specific to

the cell cycle. However, tubulin-binding agents interfere with microtubules, which are used to form spindle fibers during the mitotic phase of the cell cycle. If the spindle fibers are disrupted, chromosome alignment cannot happen properly and cell division will be halted.

6. **The correct answer is A.** Stem cells that originate in the bone marrow serve as the precursor to all blood cells. These include the erythrocytes, leukocytes, and platelets. If a person has leukemia and abnormal leukocytes, a stem cell transplant would allow for the differentiation of new and hopefully normal leukocytes. Stem cells do not have the ability to directly attack other cells, replace the function of abnormal cells, or act as immune system modulators.

7. **The correct answer is C.** Solutions that are hypotonic contain less solute and more water than what they are being compared to. In this case, the excess water in the extracellular fluid makes it hypotonic to the cells. This causes water to move into the cells by osmosis. Isotonic solutions have equal solute concentrations both inside and outside the cell. Hypertonic solutions have more solute and less water relative to what they are being compared to. In this case, the intracellular fluid would be hypertonic.

8. **The correct answer is A.** Sodium has a variety of roles in the body. Of the choices listed, sodium is highly involved with the function of neurons. The sodium/potassium pumps maintain an unequal balance of ions across the membrane of neurons during resting potential. During action potential, sodium channels open in order to initiate an impulse. If the sodium ion concentration is out of balance, the neuron function could be compromised.

9. **The correct answer is A.** In this case, administering a solution that is hypertonic to the cells would help. A hypertonic extracellular solution would draw water out of the swollen cells to counteract the effects of water intoxication. An isotonic solution would not help. A solution low in solute concentration would be high in water relative to the cells making the solution hypotonic, which would cause more water to enter the cells. A saline solution would be high in solutes and hypertonic to the cells.

10. **The correct answer is B.** With an extreme increase in water consumption, the plasma and blood volume increases, increasing blood pressure. The kidneys try to deal with this by increasing their filtration rate and increasing urine production to try to eliminate some of the excess water and reduce blood volume and pressure. What should not happen in this situation is to increase the retention of water in the body. Antidiuretic hormone (ADH) normally increases water reabsorption in the nephron. You would expect the secretion of ADH to drop in this circumstance so that more water can be excreted by the kidneys.

11. **The correct answer is B.** In the proximal convoluted tubule, the primary events are the reabsorption of nutrients and water. There are two regions in the nephron

where large amounts of sodium and water are reabsorbed. In the loop of Henle, the countercurrent multiplier system is used, which leads to the reabsorption of salts (sodium and chloride) and water. In the distal convoluted tubule, the hormone aldosterone influences the reabsorption of salts and water followed by osmosis.

12. **The correct answer is D.** This question relies on an understanding of the functions of brain structures. The cerebrum is involved in sensory processing, motor coordination, and association. The spinal cord relays messages to and from the brain and can process some reflex actions. The cerebellum deals with sensory-motor coordination, balance, and complex muscle movement patterns. The medulla oblongata is located in the brain stem; it has reflex centers for vital functions such as ventilation. Damage to the medulla oblongata could potentially be fatal.

13. **The correct answer is A.** The passage explains that Sertoli cells influence spermatogenesis. Therefore, the more Sertoli cells, theoretically, the more sperm should be produced. The two groups of men in this study varied in their sperm count. We are told that group 1 subjects had a normal sperm count while group 2 participants were seeking infertility treatments due to a low sperm count. Based on this information, the men with the higher sperm count should have a higher number of Sertoli cells. This would be group 1.

14. **The correct answer is B.** There are many relationships that could be deduced from these data. Keep in mind that the question says to consider the data from both groups, so we are looking for trends that are similar in groups 1 and 2. Choice A suggests a positive feedback relationship between FSH and LH. This would mean that as one of these hormones increases, so does the other. While this might be possible based on the group 1 data, it is not seen in the group 2 data. Choice C suggests a positive feedback relationship between testosterone and FSH. While this might be plausible for group 2 subjects, it is not for group 1 subjects. This leaves choice B. There is in fact a negative feedback relationship between inhibin-B and FSH. In groups 1 and 2, when inhibin-B was high, FSH was low. This suggests negative feedback. Since there is a relationship between some of these hormones, choice D can be eliminated.

15. **The correct answer is C.** The passage explains that group 1 men have normal sperm counts while group 2 men have low sperm counts. In looking at the data, the testosterone levels between groups 1 and 2 are not significantly different, which indicates that this hormone is not a good indicator of sperm count. The LH data for both groups tend to be fairly low and not drastically different between the groups. For FSH, the level is higher in the group 2 men who have a lower sperm count. Inhibin-B is the only feasible option as it is high in the men with normal sperm counts and low in the men with low sperm counts.

16. **The correct answer is A.** The blood-testis barrier is described in the passage as a barricade to establish immune privilege for the testes. To answer this question,

you need to think about how the sperm cells in the testes would compare to other cells in the body. Sperm cells are haploid, and all are genetically different from each other and from other cells in the body. Because they are genetically different, they should express unique surface antigens. If the cells of the immune system were to contact the sperm, they would be perceived as foreign and could be subject to immune system attack, which would destroy the sperm. For this reason, the blood-testes barrier is required to keep the sperm away from the immune cells. The remaining choices do not make good sense. Sperm cells will eventually leave the reproductive system during ejaculation. It also would not make sense to indicate that the blood flow to the testes needs to be cut off. This would prevent oxygen and nutrient flow to the area. Preventing the sperm from moving to the epididymis before they are ready does not provide an explanation for why the sperm cells need to be kept separate from the cells of the immune system.

17. **The correct answer is B.** This question relies on your knowledge of the female reproductive cycle. In women, as FSH levels climb, follicles are stimulated to grow. These follicles produce estrogen, which exerts positive feedback on LH, whose levels begin to climb. When LH levels peak on the 14th day of the cycle, the follicle ruptures, releasing the egg from the ovary and leaving the corpus luteum behind in the ovary. After ovulation, the corpus luteum secretes both estrogen and progesterone to inhibit GnRH. When GnRH is inhibited, FSH and LH will also be inhibited. Choice B correctly indicates that the LH surge causes ovulation.

18. **The correct answer is A.** This question relies on your knowledge of cell division. Mitosis is the process by which differentiated cells produce identical daughter cells.

19. **The correct answer is C.** For species C, the comparison of brain size and testes size relative to body weight is approximately equal. In species A, the relative testes size is much bigger than brain size, which indicates the females are more promiscuous in this group. In species B, the relative brain size is larger than testes size, indicating that the females are monogamous. The best explanation for species C having a fairly equal balance between relative brain and testes sizes is that the females are not completely monogamous, nor are they polygamous.

20. **The correct answer is C.** Decreasing the overall weight of the bat would not necessarily indicate that there was more energy to be devoted to sperm production. While it might be plausible that smaller bats can avoid predation, other species of bats have not decreased in weight and have managed to survive. We have no indication or evidence that smaller males can mate more easily. Choice C is the most logical of the choices given by suggesting that lighter animals have flight advantages.

21. **The correct answer is A.** Natural selection allows for the most fit organisms to reproduce more, passing on their genes to the next generation. Over many

generations, allelic frequencies change in the population. From a fitness perspective, all that matters is reproducing. How healthy, intelligent, or robust a bat is doesn't matter if it doesn't reproduce and pass on its genes. The males who have larger testes produce more sperm and reproduce more.

22. **The correct answer is A.** If the data from the bat study could be related to primates (which is not necessarily possible), we would expect that chimpanzees would have relatively large testes at the expense of a small brain. Gorillas should have relatively smaller testes allowing for more energy to be focused on larger brains. Of the choices given, choice A is most accurate. Chimpanzees would have larger testes and smaller brains (less intelligence) than gorillas.

23. **The correct answer is B.** Fitness is completely relative. The most fit individuals reproduce more and pass on their genes to the next generation. Being large and healthy does not imply anything about your ability to reproduce and pass on your genes. Further, being smart and avoiding predation does not necessarily mean that your genes get passed on to the next generation. A male with large testes who can make a lot of sperm and reproduce frequently would be considered the most fit of the choices given.

24. **The correct answer is D.** Artificial selection would suggest that something other than natural factors selected for the trait of large testes. In stabilizing selection, an intermediate phenotype is favored, which would cause the increase in phenotype of males with average-sized testes. In disruptive selection, the two extreme phenotypes are favored equally. This would produce males with either very small or very large testes. In directional selection, one extreme phenotype is favored—in this case, males with large testes.

25. **The correct answer is C.** Death of osteoblasts due to *S. aureus* infection is the result of induction of apoptosis. Apoptosis is triggered by capsase-8, so increasing the activity of capsase-8 would increase the rate of apoptosis and osteoblast death. Further, capsase-8 is activated by TRAIL made by *S. aureus,* so increasing the TRAIL activity would also increase osteoblast death rates. A drug that is antagonistic to TRAIL would decrease capsase-8 activity and decrease the rate of apoptosis in osteoblasts.

26. **The correct answer is D.** The leukocytes that engulf microbes such as bacteria are macrophages. This process is termed *phagocytosis*. Basophils secrete histamine, which is involved in the initiation of the inflammatory response. Lymphocytes are involved in specific immune system defenses. Eosinophils are involved in the defense response to antigens from unique sources such as parasites.

27. **The correct answer is C.** Complement proteins circulate in the blood in an inactive form. When bacteria enter the blood, the complement proteins are activated, which causes a cascade of reactions that ultimately cause lysis and death of the bacteria. Antibody production or cytotoxic T-cell activation could certainly

be stimulated by bacteria in the blood, but the question stipulated that this must be a nonspecific defense and these defenses are specific. Interleukins are cytokines secreted by immune cells, and they would not directly be able to defend against bacteria in the bloodstream.

28. **The correct answer is B.** Bacteria spontaneously mutate in order to produce diversity in the population. Some bacteria have spontaneous mutations, usually on plasmids, that allow them to survive in the presence of certain antibiotics. If the bacterial population is repeatedly exposed to that antibiotic due to overuse, it exerts selective pressure where only the resistant bacteria survive. These resistant bacteria multiply, and in the next generation a higher frequency of resistance is observed. Antibiotic resistance has nothing to do with people becoming resistant to antibiotics—it is all about the bacterial mutations.

29. **The correct answer is C.** This question relies on your knowledge of bacterial cell structures and functions. The nucleoid is the region of the cell where the one circular loop of chromosomal DNA is located. The ribosomes are responsible for protein synthesis. Bacteria can convert themselves to spores when environmental conditions are poor, allowing them to survive for extended periods of time in harsh conditions. The capsule is a sticky layer surrounding the cell that helps in the attachment of the cell to a surface. It is likely that the adhesins are located here.

30. **The correct answer is A.** Knowledge of the endocrine structures and hormones is needed to answer this question. The hormone calcitonin stimulates the storage of calcium in bone matrix. Its target is the osteoblasts that build new bone matrix. The calcitonin hormone is made by the thyroid gland. Parathyroid hormone is antagonistic to calcitonin and stimulates osteoclasts. Osteotonin is not a real hormone.

31. **The correct answer is D.** Based on the data given, drug Y is the only treatment to show a mean decrease in pulmonary artery pressure, which is the goal of this experiment. While some individual patients in the drug X and placebo groups did show a decrease in pulmonary artery pressure, the overall results for these groups included an increase in mean pulmonary artery pressure.

32. **The correct answer is B.** The results from the drug X group indicate that the treatment caused an increase in mean pulmonary artery pressure. This helps us to eliminate choice A, which suggests that drug X is binding to ETA. If this were the case, the drug would be bound to ETA so that endothelin could only bind to ETB. When endothelin binds to ETB, vasodilation occurs, implying a decrease in pressure. This was not seen in the drug X group. Choice B suggests that drug X is selectively binding to the ETB receptor. This would mean that endothelin could only bind to ETA, which does in fact cause an increase in pressure. This would be the correct choice.

33. **The correct answer is C.** To answer this question, you must be familiar with the anatomy of the heart. The right side of the heart is the pulmonary circuit while the left side is the systemic circuit. Deoxygenated blood enters the right atrium of the heart via the superior and inferior vena cava. Blood from the right atrium passes through the tricuspid valve to the right ventricle and then leaves the heart through the pulmonary semilunar valve. Blood is carried via the pulmonary arteries to the lungs where gas exchange occurs. After gas exchange occurs, oxygenated blood returns to the heart via pulmonary veins to enter the left atrium. From there blood passes through the bicuspid valve into the left ventricle. Blood leaves the left side of the heart by passing through the aortic valve into the aorta. If there was a pressure increase in the pulmonary arteries, the right ventricle of the heart would be most likely affected as it is the last chamber that blood is located in before it moves toward the lungs in the pulmonary arteries.

34. **The correct answer is B.** Overexpression of the ETB receptor means that endothelin will have more ETB receptors to bind to. The passage indicated that when endothelin binds to the ETB receptor, vasodilation occurs, which decreases blood pressure. This would suggest that the patient's blood pressure would decrease, the explanation provided by choice B.

35. **The correct answer is A.** This question expects you to be able to consider how the kidneys are involved in regulating blood volume and blood pressure. Water that is reabsorbed in the nephrons returns to the bloodstream to increase plasma volume, which in turn increases blood pressure as the volume of blood increases. When the nephrons absorb more water to increase blood volume, the urine volume decreases. The two hormones aldosterone and antidiuretic hormone help increase the amount of water reabsorbed by nephrons, which in turn decreases urine volume. In order to reduce blood pressure, the kidneys can decrease the amount of water reabsorbed by the nephrons. The less water reabsorbed means there will be less blood volume and less blood pressure. This would ultimately increase urine volume. The question asks how the kidneys might try to reduce hypertension. This would mean that we want less water reabsorbed into the blood, which would decrease blood volume and blood pressure. To do this, urine volume would have to increase.

36. **The correct answer is B.** The question suggests that ETA can be activated by certain types of endothelin, which causes ETA to synergize with growth factors to increase cell proliferation rates. Growth factors are one of many mechanisms used to regulate the cell cycle. Of the choices listed, A, C, and D can be eliminated as they have nothing to do with growth factors and cell proliferation. The only reasonable answer is choice B since one of the many characteristics of cancer is increased cell proliferation.

37. **The correct answer is C.** The data report estrogen concentration. From reviewing the data, it can be seen that the mutant strain generally has a higher estrogen concentration than the wild type strain.

38. **The correct answer is D.** Rate-limiting steps generally require the highest activation energies and are the slowest steps in a metabolic pathway.

39. **The correct answer is C.** Estrogen levels typically peak prior to ovulation, triggering the LH surge that is responsible for ovulation. For this reason, we would see the highest levels of estrogen around the time of ovulation, which should lead to a decrease in total and LDL cholesterol levels at that time.

40. **The correct answer is A.** One primary role of cholesterol is to stabilize the plasma membrane and to regulate fluidity of the membrane.

41. **The correct answer is C.** Because the mutant mice have a higher estrogen level due to the mutation in the rate-limiting step, it is likely that their cholesterol levels will be lower. Since cholesterol is converted to estrogen, if that process is occurring more rapidly than normal, the cholesterol levels may be lower than normal since the cholesterol is being converted to estrogen.

42. **The correct answer is D.** In the mutant mice, cholesterol is converted to estrogen at a faster rate. We would expect sexually mature mice to have a reduced cholesterol level due to estrogen production as compared to a mouse that is not close to sexual maturity.

43. **The correct answer is B.** The passage explains that estrogen seems to provide some sort of protective role against HIV infection. There is no mention of the role of testosterone with this hypothesis, so we should assume that it is not important to this theory. Therefore, choices A and D can be eliminated. Choice C introduces the idea of a female who has had her ovaries removed. Since the ovaries produce estrogen, assume that this female's estrogen levels would be decreased. Based on the information in the passage, this female should have less protection against HIV infection due to the decreased estrogen levels. Choice B introduces a female who oversecretes estrogen. Since the passage tells us that estrogen provides some protection against HIV infection, this female should be the most likely candidate (of the choices listed) to be protected against HIV infection.

44. **The correct answer is A.** This question requires you to know some of the details of the female reproductive cycle including what hormones are involved following ovulation. Prior to ovulation, both follicle stimulating hormone (FSH) and luteinizing hormone (LH) are secreted from the anterior pituitary and are involved in follicular growth and maturation. The secretion of both FSH and LH is stimulated by gonadotropin-releasing hormone (GnRH) from the hypothalamus. As the follicles grow and mature, they produce estrogen. During the second week of the cycle, increasing estrogen levels cause a spike in LH levels, which causes ovulation. Recall that following ovulation, the remnant of the follicle that stays in the

ovary is called the corpus luteum. The corpus luteum secretes both estrogen and progesterone, which inhibit the further release of FSH and LH. The question is asking about a unique hormone that causes increased risk of HIV following ovulation. Choices B and D can be eliminated because FSH and LH are hormones most active prior to ovulation. Choice C is not appropriate since estrogen is secreted prior to and following ovulation. The only hormone that is unique to postovulation is progesterone, which makes choice A correct.

45. **The correct answer is A.** Since CCR5 is a coreceptor for HIV, up-regulation of the CCR5 allele should provide more receptors for HIV making it more likely for more cells to become infected as is indicated by choice A. The remaining choices are not reasonable explanations. Since increased expression of CCR5 should make it easier for cells to become infected, choice B would not be plausible. Choice C does not provide an adequate explanation, particularly since the passage indicates that while in the earlier phases of infection, women carry higher lower loads than men. The passage also indicates that the delta-32 allele of CCR5 provides protection against HIV infection, not the normal CCR5 allele, which eliminates choice D.

46. **The correct answer is B.** To answer this question, you need to rely on your knowledge of genetics. The passage states that the delta-32 CCR5 mutation is protective against HIV infection. The question indicated that there are two different phenotypes noted within the delta-32 CCR5 mutation—one that offers near 100% protection against HIV infection and one that offers only partial protection. The best explanation for why two phenotypes (complete protection and partial protection) are observed would be that the delta-32 allele exhibits incomplete dominance. An individual that is homozygous for the allele (meaning he or she inherited two copies of the delta-32 allele) would have full protection, while an individual who is heterozygous (meaning he or she has one normal copy of the allele and one copy of the delta-32 allele) would have an intermediate phenotype (being partial protection). This is indicated by choice B. Since the question indicates that the differences in phenotype (protection) are related to the delta-32 mutation, choices A and D can be eliminated as they suppose that something other than the allele is providing protection. Choice C suggests that epistasis is involved in masking the delta-32 allele. While this might sound remotely plausible, choice B is a much more likely explanation.

47. **The correct answer is C.** You need to know what retroviruses are and have a basic understanding of how they operate to answer this question. Retroviruses have the unique ability to transcribe their RNA to DNA (recall that the central dogma indicates DNA to RNA to protein) so that the viral genetic material can integrate into host cell chromosomes to initiate the latent phase of the life cycle. In order to transcribe the RNA to DNA, the enzyme reverse transcriptase is needed, which is indicated by choice C. The other choices relate to enzymes that are not specific

to retroviruses. DNA polymerase is used by cells to copy DNA during the process of semiconservative replication. RNA polymerase is used by cells to perform the conversion of DNA to RNA (transcription). Helicase is the enzyme in cells that is used to unwind the DNA double helix.

48. **The correct answer is D.** The question explains that AZT and ddI interfere with replication and transcription. During a viral infection, the ideal situation would be to interfere with viral processes while leaving host cell processes unaffected. Choice A suggests that host cell DNA replication should be prevented in order to keep the host cell from functioning and mentions nothing about how this would affect the virus. Choice B is similar in that it does not mention how the virus would be affected. Choice C is not appropriate because it discusses preventing infection. If the patient is already confirmed as infected, then this choice wouldn't make sense. If a person is infected with HIV, then the viral genetic material has already entered the host cells. If replication of the viral genome can be prevented as suggested by choice D, then the progression of the infection can be slowed.

49. **The correct answer is B.** From the graph provided, it seems that culturable bacteria decreased significantly (almost to 0) during the course of antibiotic therapy, which indicates that the antibiotic treatment was successful at eliminating culturable bacteria. However, the number of nonculturable but metabolically active cells stayed approximately equal during the course of the antibiotic therapy, which suggests that those cells did not respond to the treatment. This eliminates choice A as a possible answer since not all *E. coli* were eliminated by antibiotic treatment. The culturable bacteria causing the infection were eliminated by antibiotic treatment, which removes choice C as a possible answer. Choice D suggests that the treatment increased the number of *E. coli*, which is in direct contrast to what is shown on the graph. The best conclusion is that while the culturable bacteria have been eliminated, the nonculturable bacteria have made the patient at risk for developing another UTI should the nonculturable bacteria resuscitate to culturable form. This is indicated by choice B.

50. **The correct answer is D.** To support the VBNC hypothesis, it is necessary to provide evidence that the cells are metabolically active. The presence of DNA, proteins, or an intact cell membrane within the cell does not necessarily provide sufficient evidence to indicate that the cells are metabolically active because these things could be found in dying or dead cells. This eliminates choices A, B, and C. However, if one could show evidence of transcription occurring within the cells, this would provide good support for the fact that they are metabolically active.

51. **The correct answer is B.** In order to answer this question, you need to be familiar with the anatomy of the male and female reproductive and urinary systems. The passage explains that the *E. coli* bacteria that are normal residents of the digestive tract can cause UTIs when they enter the urinary tract. This means that we are

looking for a difference between men and women that would allow the bacteria to move from the intestinal tract to the urinary tract. There would be no reasonable support to suggest that women have a poorer immune response than men or that the bacteria infecting women are more likely to be resistant to antibiotics. This eliminates choices C and D. The number of *E. coli* in the intestinal tract is insignificant because the only concern is whether they enter the urinary tract to cause infection, which eliminates choice A. In the anatomy of the female system, the urethra is much closer to the anus, which makes for a short traveling distance for the bacteria that are able to get to the urethra. In males, the urethra is longer and farther away from the anus, making it harder for the bacteria to get to the urethra. The anatomical difference suggested by choice B is the only reasonable explanation for why women are more likely to contract UTIs.

52. **The correct answer is D.** Based on the data provided in the figure, the best assumption is that the trends seen in the graph would continue over time. It appears that the antibiotic therapy eliminated the culturable bacteria, so it would be safe to assume that the numbers of culturable bacteria would remain very low. This would eliminate choice A, which says that culturable cell count would increase. Since the cell counts for metabolically active cells did not decrease during the initial antibiotic treatment, there is no reason to assume that they would eventually decrease over a longer period, thus eliminating choices B and C. Based on the fact that the number of nonculturable bacteria did not decrease over the time period shown, we can assume that this is unlikely to change over a longer time course. Assuming that the trends seen in the graph continue, choice D is the most appropriate prediction.

53. **The correct answer is B.** This question relies on an understanding of antibiotic resistance. The overuse of antibiotics puts pressure on bacteria that selects for the bacteria that have mutated to become resistant to antibiotics. The overuse of antibiotics eliminates the susceptible bacteria, which leaves only the resistant bacteria to multiple to large numbers. Choice A suggests that people become immune to antibiotics, which is false. Since antibiotics are designed to target bacteria, bacteria are the only things that can become resistant to antibiotics. Since antibiotics normally kill bacteria, choice D would not make sense since it suggests that the use of antibiotics would increase the populations of resident bacteria. Choice C just isn't logical. Since many antibiotics are used on a routine basis, we know that they don't typically cause massive organ damage.

54. **The correct answer is B.** If the VBNC cells were able to resuscitate to fully metabolically active cells, this would indicate that they were not in the process of dying.

55. **The correct answer is A.** This question relies on a knowledge of dominant and recessive patterns of inheritance. Dominant alleles are expressed, even in the heterozygous individual. In this case, our example is a dominant allele that causes a

fatal condition. Since every individual carrying a single allele of this type would likely not survive, we would expect the frequency of the allele to decrease over time. In contrast, disorders that follow recessive patterns of inheritance require two copies of the allele for expression. Those who are heterozygous do not express the disorder and thus would survive.

56. **The correct answer is B.** Antibodies are proteins that are secreted from the cell. Proteins would be produced and labeled by the rough endoplasmic reticulum. From there, they would be sorted by the Golgi complex and finally directed to the cell membrane for secretion.

57. **The correct answer is B.** This question relies on a knowledge of the basic chemical composition of the biologically important molecules. Carbohydrates and lipids are composed of C, O, and H. However, DNA is a nucleic acid and contains phosphate groups.

58. **The correct answer is A.** This question is asking how to move a potassium ion (which is small) from an area that has a low concentration to an area with a relatively higher concentration. In this case we are moving against the concentration gradient. The transport type that could do this is active transport, using energy to move the ions against their concentration gradient.

59. **The correct answer is C.** During the electron transport chain, oxygen serves as the terminal electron acceptor during aerobic respiration. In addition to serving as an electron acceptor, the oxygen also gathers protons from the electron transport chain, producing water in the process.

60. **The correct answer is C.** This question relies on your knowledge of semiconservative DNA replication where a single double helix is separated in order for both strands of the double helix to serve as templates for the production of new strands.

61. **The correct answer is A.** Of the choices presented, the only accurate choice is A. DNA nucleotides utilize the sugar deoxyribose while RNA nucleotides utilize the sugar ribose. Of the remaining choices, B is incorrect because we know that DNA uses T nucleotides while RNA uses U nucleotides. Choice C is not correct because RNA is produced in transcription and a protein is produced in translation. Finally, choice D is incorrect because DNA is double-stranded and RNA is single-stranded.

62. **The correct answer is C.** In order to answer this question you need to recall the human diploid number of 46. In mitosis, a diploid parent cell produces two diploid daughter cells.

63. **The correct answer is C.** Steroid hormones exert their effects by entering into cells and binding with a receptor in the cytoplasm. The hormone-receptor complex then enters the nucleus where it acts to alter gene expression in the cell. Since the question is asking about nonsteroid, or peptide, hormones, choices A and B can be eliminated. Choice D can also be eliminated as this is not a plausible explanation. Nonsteroid hormones act as first messengers, binding to their receptors on the

cell membrane. The hormone itself does not enter the cell. The binding of the first messenger to the receptor causes a series of reaction in the cell that ultimately activate second messengers, such as cAMP.

64. **The correct answer is A.** RNA polymerase binds to the promoter site on the DNA template, at which time it is free to begin transcription. The regulator gene is a type of control gene that produces a small protein called a repressor. The operon is a group of linked genes composed of the operator and its adjacent structural genes.

65. **The correct answer is C.** During anaerobic respiration, glycolysis and fermentation occur. The process of fermentation does not produce ATP. The only ATP made during anaerobic respiration is from glycolysis. The net gain of ATP in glycolysis per molecule of ATP is two. If the cell has access to six molecules of glucose and each molecule will produce 2 ATP, then a total of 12 ATP will be produced.

Section 2. Chemical and Physical Foundations of Biological Systems

1. **The correct answer is B.** As described in the passage, treatment of olefins with acid results in a carbocationic intermediate, which is prone to shifts and rearrangements. In this case, a hydride shift is very facile, the driving force being the conversion of a secondary cation into a tertiary variety. Subsequent capture of the electrophilic center with water, followed by proton transfer, leads to Product B.

2. **The correct answer is A.** As described in the passage, the use of mercuric ion prevents the formation of a formal carbocation, and therefore suppresses rearrangements. The intermediate mercurinium ion is captured by water at either secondary position to give an organomercury compound, which is demercurated with sodium borohydride to give Product A.

3. **The correct answer is B.** Product B is the only product with symmetry (specifically, an internal mirror plane); therefore, there are two sets of carbon atoms related by symmetry, which give rise to only one signal for each set. The other three products lack this symmetry element and are expected to exhibit peaks for all eight carbons in the skeleton.

4. **The correct answer is A.** There are two chiral centers and the molecule is chiral. Both the *cis*- and *trans*-isomers have two chiral centers (the tertiary centers are connected to four different groups); however, the *cis*-isomer possesses a mirror plane that destroys the chirality on a molecular level. In other words, the *cis*-isomer is a *meso* compound. The *trans*-isomer lacks this symmetry element and thus is classified as a chiral molecule.

5. **The correct answer is A.** The demercuration step involves the attack of hydride on the carbon bearing the mercury, resulting in a net $2e^-$ reduction from Hg^{2+} to Hg^0, as shown:

6. **The correct answer is C.** As noted in the text of the problem, the flying bird is subject to four forces: weight, drag, lift, and thrust. Since the bird has mass, it is subject to the force due to gravity or weight, which acts straight downward. Thus, choice B can be eliminated. Drag is the air resistance force encountered in flight, a force that acts opposite to the direction of flight motion. Since the bird in the diagram is moving to the left, drag is a force represented by an arrow directed to the left. This is provided by choice C, the correct choice. Lift is an upward directed force, and thrust is the pushing force acting to propel the bird in the direction of its motion—to the left.

7. **The correct answer is C.** The blood's volumetric flow rate, Q, is related to flow velocity, v, by the following relation:

$$Q = vA$$

where A is the cross-sectional area of the blood vessel. The volumetric flow rate must first be converted to units of $\dfrac{cm^3}{s}$:

$$Q = 5\frac{L}{min} \times \frac{1000\,cm^3}{1\,L} \times \frac{1\,min}{60\,s} = 83.3\frac{cm^3}{s}$$

The cross-sectional area of the vessel, A, is:

$$A = \pi r^2 = (3.14)(1.2\,cm)^2 = 4.52\,cm^2$$

Thus, the blood flow velocity is:

$$v = \frac{83.3\frac{cm^3}{s}}{4.52\,cm^2} = 18.4\frac{cm}{s}$$

8. **The correct answer is A.** The current, I, is related to the amount of charge, Δq, that flows during a time interval, Δt, by:

$$I = \frac{\Delta q}{\Delta t} \Rightarrow \Delta q = I \cdot \Delta t = (15\,A)(0.007\,s) = 0.105\,C$$

9. **The correct answer is C.** Because the steps of the reaction and the listed heats of reaction are exactly aligned to how the reaction takes place, there is no need to

switch any reactions or reverse any signs for the heats of reaction. This allows you to simply add up the heats of reaction: $+92 +121 +496 -349 -771 = -411$ kJ.

10. **The correct answer is B.** The chloride ion has 18 electrons now that it has gained an electron. The new configuration will show a stable octet in the 3s and 3p orbitals combined: $1s^2 2s^2 2p^6 3s^2 3p^6$.

11. **The correct answer is B.** The lattice energy increases with increasing charge. Clearly the negative two charge of sulfur is greater. Also, sulfur is about the same size as chlorine, meaning that for the (almost) same size ions, the sulfur has double the negative charge.

12. **The correct answer is A.** The lattice energy is always a positive value, eliminating choices B and D. The lattice energy is also the formation of the solid lattice structure from the gaseous ions, the fifth elementary step. Finally, looking at the chart you see that LiCl and KCl have their values listed. Using periodic trends and relationships, the lattice energy for NaCl should fall in between those of LiCl and KCl.

13. **The correct answer is C.** The stable sodium element has 11 protons in the nucleus and 11 orbiting electrons. The sodium ion lacks one electron needed for stability, giving it an overall positive charge of $+1$. The correct Lewis structure for the sodium ion is Na^+.

14. **The correct answer is A.** When heat energy is absorbed, the electrons enter a higher energy state. Light is emitted when the electrons fall back to the ground state.

15. **The correct answer is C.** This question can be solved using the lens equation:

$$\frac{1}{\text{object distance}} + \frac{1}{\text{image distance}} = \frac{1}{\text{focal length}}$$

The reader can substitute the values for object distance and focal length from each option into the above equation and solve for the image distance which, for Lens Scenario 3, yields:

$$\frac{1}{\text{image distance}} = \frac{1}{\text{focal length}} - \frac{1}{\text{object distance}} = \frac{1}{f} - \frac{1}{f} = 0$$

which implies an undefined image. The solution could also be determined by drawing a ray diagram.

16. **The correct answer is D.** This problem can be solved using the lens equation:

$$\frac{1}{\text{object distance}} + \frac{1}{\text{image distance}} = \frac{1}{\text{focal length}}$$

The reader can substitute the values for object distance and focal length from each option into the above equation and Lens Scenario 4 yields:

$$\frac{1}{\text{image distance}} = \frac{1}{\text{focal length}} - \frac{1}{\text{object distance}}$$

$$= \frac{1}{f} - \frac{1}{f/2} = \frac{1}{f} - \frac{2}{f} = -\frac{1}{f}$$

In other words, image distance = – focal length. A negative image distance implies a virtual image, which is always upright. The solution could also be determined by drawing a ray diagram.

17. **The correct answer is C.** This question can be solved using the lens equation:

$$\frac{1}{\text{object distance}} + \frac{1}{\text{image distance}} = \frac{1}{\text{focal length}}$$

Substituting the values for object distance and focal length from Lens Scenario 2:

$$\frac{1}{\text{image distance}} = \frac{1}{\text{focal length}} - \frac{1}{\text{object distance}}$$

$$= \frac{1}{f} - \frac{1}{2f} = \frac{2}{2f} - \frac{1}{2f} = \frac{1}{2f}$$

In other words, image distance = 2f, given by choice C.

18. **The correct answer is A.** The image magnification, m, can be determined from the equation:

$$m = -\frac{\text{image distance}}{\text{object distance}}$$

One first needs to determine the image distance for Lens Scenario 1 by using the lens equation:

$$\frac{1}{\text{object distance}} + \frac{1}{\text{image distance}} = \frac{1}{\text{focal length}}$$

Substituting the values for object distance and focal length from Lens Scenario 1:

$$\frac{1}{\text{image distance}} = \frac{1}{\text{focal length}} - \frac{1}{\text{object distance}}$$

$$= \frac{1}{f} - \frac{1}{3f} = \frac{3}{3f} - \frac{1}{3f} = \frac{2}{3f}$$

In other words, image distance = $\frac{3f}{2}$ cm. Substituting the information provided for Lens Scenario 1 yields:

$$m = -\frac{\text{image distance}}{\text{object distance}} = -\frac{\frac{3f}{2}\text{cm}}{3f \text{ cm}} = -\frac{1}{2}$$

The fact that m is negative implies that the image is inverted with respect to the object. The value of $\frac{1}{2}$ implies that is smaller than the object or reduced by 2.

19. **The correct answer is A.** One first starts with the lens equation and then solving for the focal length, f:

$$\frac{1}{\text{focal length}} = \frac{1}{\text{object distance}} + \frac{1}{\text{image distance}}$$

$$= \frac{\text{image distance} + \text{object distance}}{(\text{object distance})(\text{image distance})}$$

Thus, the focal length is:

$$\text{focal length} = \frac{(\text{object distance})\,(\text{image distance})}{\text{image distance} + \text{object distance}}$$

20. **The correct answer is C.** The molecule in the box is already in an eclipsed conformation required for a Fischer projection. Therefore, since the bromines are on opposite sides in the dash-wedge projection, they must also be on opposite sides in the Fischer, and we can exclude choices A and D. The remaining choices (B and C) are enantiomeric—distinguishing between the two is best carried out by imagining a vantage point from above the dash-wedge representation, as shown:

It is then apparent that the upper bromine would point to the right and the lower bromine would be directed to the left of the observer.

21. **The correct answer is D.**

The chemical transformation involves a Jones oxidation of the primary alcohol to form a carboxylic acid, followed by treatment with diazomethane to form the methyl ester, as shown:

The stereochemistry of the chiral center has not changed; its identity to the given product can be shown by a vertical flip:

22. **The correct answer is D.** The product is an alkene without optical activity. The starting material, (*S*)-2-chloro-4-methylpentane, possesses a good leaving group on a secondary center with adjacent protons. Therefore, all four common pathways (S_N1, S_N2, E1, and E2) are available to it. However, potassium *tert*-butoxide is a strong hindered base that is unlikely to engage in substitution reactions

(i.e., favors elimination). Once the elimination occurs, the chiral center is destroyed; therefore, the product cannot exhibit optical activity.

23. **The correct answer is C.** Choice A shows the wrong formula for calcium hydroxide, and choice B is not correctly balanced. Choice D shows calcium ion reacting, instead of the appropriate calcium metal. The complete, balanced equation is choice C.

24. **The correct answer is A.** Looking at the series, K and Na will react with water as they are very reactive metals. Only calcium, strontium, and barium from Group 2 *do* react with water. Mg does not and is the first in the series *not* to react with water.

25. **The correct answer is C.** Cobalt is more reactive than the copper and less reactive than iron. This puts the activity of copper between the two. There is no basis from the passage to compare cobalt's activity to that of lead.

26. **The correct answer is D.** Nickel is better at losing electrons than silver. Therefore, silver ions will attract electrons from nickel and become solid silver. Only copper, silver, and gold will be resistant to acid from the series. Chromium will react with acid. Calcium is better at losing electrons than aluminum. Therefore, aluminum ions will attract electrons from calcium and become solid aluminum. Choice D is false because tin has a lesser tendency to lose electrons than nickel.

27. **The correct answer is B.** Chromium has 24 electrons, and it has one of the anomalous electron configurations of $1s^2 2s^2 2p^6 3s^2 3p^6 \underline{3d^5 4s^1}$.

28. **The correct answer is D.** A diamagnetic element is characterized by the fact that all of its electrons are paired. Of the four choices, the only metal that fits this description is copper.

29. **The correct answer is B.** The number of neutrons is the mass number A minus the atomic number Z. Thus, the number of neutrons of iodine-131 is $N = A - Z = 131 - 53 = 78$.

30. **The correct answer is A.** The weight of an object or a substance can be calculated using the following equation:

$$W = mg$$

Weight = (mass)(acceleration due to gravity)

To find the mass of the blood sample, one uses the density equation:

$$\rho = \frac{m}{V}$$

where ρ = density, m = mass, and V = volume. Given in the problem are the density of blood ($\rho = 1.06 \, \text{g/cm}^3$) and the volume of blood ($V = 10 \, \text{mL} = 10 \, \text{cm}^3$).

Rearranging the above equation for mass and substituting known values yields:

$$m = \rho V = (1.06\,\text{g/cm}^3)\,(10\,\text{cm}^3). = 10.6\,\text{g}$$

However, in order to substitute into the equation for weight, mass must be expressed in terms of kilograms, not grams, which results in 0.0106 kg. Thus, $W = (0.0106\,\text{kg})\,(9.8\,\text{m/s}^2) = 0.104\,\text{N}$.

31. **The correct answer is C.** Sulfur is lower on the periodic table, therefore methyl thiolate is both more polarizable (thus, more nucleophilic) and larger (less basic).

32. **The correct answer is D.** Just as sulfur is lower on the periodic table than oxygen, iodine is lower than chlorine; therefore, iodide is more polarizable and more nucleophilic than chloride. The same top-to-bottom trend makes iodide less basic than chloride. Neither is terribly basic; nevertheless, inasmuch as chloride is the stronger base (i.e., weaker conjugate acid), it is the poorer leaving group.

33. **The correct answer is C.** Methyl thiolate is the stronger nucleophile; iodide is the better leaving group. Therefore, the most favorable reaction will be between those two species.

34. **The correct answer is C.** Increasing temperature always increases rate. The rate enhancement for elimination will be greater because of entropy effects, but both processes will be faster.

35. **The correct answer is B.** Methanol is a polar protic solvent, which tends to retard S_N2 by strongly coordinating to the nucleophile. Ether and THF are not protic, but they are only moderately polar. Dimethylsulfoxide (DMSO) is a very polar aprotic solvent, which coordinates cations very effectively but leaves the anion "naked" and more prone to engage in nucleophilic attack.

36. **The correct answer is B.** Before you can draw a free-body diagram representing the mass, you must first identify the forces acting on the mass. Because the object has mass, it has weight that acts downward. In addition, because the mass is attached to a string, the string exerts a force of tension through the string, directed upward. The free-body diagram that correctly represents these forces in magnitude and direction is the diagram depicted in choice B.

37. **The correct answer is A.** In order to determine the acceleration of the system, one must apply Newton's second law to each of the two masses in Atwood's machine. Since each mass is moving in the y-direction:

$$m_1: \quad \sum F_y = ma_y \qquad m_2: \quad \sum F_y = ma_y$$

$$T - m_1 g = m_1 a \qquad\qquad m_2 g - T = m_2 a$$

$$T = m_1 a + m_1 g \qquad\qquad T = m_2 g - m_2 a$$

Setting the two expressions for the tension, T, equal to one another yields:

$$m_1 a + m_1 g = m_2 g - m_2 a$$

Solving for a yields:

$$a = \frac{(m_2 - m_1)}{(m_1 + m_2)} g$$

38. **The correct answer is C.** The information given in the problem was that Atwood's machine has $m_1 = 140\,\text{g}$ and $m_2 = 160\,\text{g}$. As was shown in the solution to the previous problem, the tension expressed in terms of either of the masses is:

$$T = m_1 a + m_1 g \quad \text{or} \quad T = m_2 g - m_2 a$$

Either expression can be used, but the acceleration of the system needs to be determined. The general expression for the acceleration (which was the basis for the previous problem) is:

$$a = \frac{(m_2 - m_1)}{(m_1 + m_2)} g$$

Substituting given values:

$$a = \frac{(0.16\,\text{kg} - 0.14\,\text{kg})}{(0.14\,\text{kg} + 0.16\,\text{kg})} \left(9.8 \frac{m}{s^2}\right) = 0.65 \frac{m}{s^2}$$

Substituting into the equation in terms of m_1:

$$T = m_1 a + m_1 g = (0.14\,\text{kg})\left(0.65 \frac{m}{s^2}\right) + (0.14\,\text{kg})\left(9.8 \frac{m}{s^2}\right)$$

$$= 0.091\,\text{N} + 1.372\,\text{N} = 1.46\,\text{N}$$

You could also substitute into the equation in terms of m_2 and obtain the same result for T:

$$T = m_2 g - m_2 a = (0.16\,\text{kg})\left(9.8 \frac{m}{s^2}\right) - (0.16\,\text{kg})\left(0.65 \frac{m}{s^2}\right)$$

$$= 1.568\,\text{N} - 0.104\,\text{N} = 1.46\,\text{N}$$

39. **The correct answer is D.** The expression for the acceleration (determined in the second problem of this set) is:

$$a = \frac{(m_2 - m_1)}{(m_1 + m_2)} g$$

where $m_1 = 80$ g and $m_2 = 220$ g. Substituting all given values:

$$a = \frac{(0.22 \text{ kg} - 0.08 \text{ kg})}{(0.08 \text{ kg} + 0.22 \text{ kg})} \left(9.8 \frac{m}{s^2}\right) = 4.57 \frac{m}{s^2}$$

40. **The correct answer is A.** To determine an expression for the tension in Atwood's machine, you can begin with the same two equations of motion for the two masses derived from Newton's second law of motion or:

$$m_1: T - m_1 g = m_1 a \quad m_2: m_2 g - T = m_2 a$$

Solving both equations for the acceleration, a, yields:

$$m_1: a = \frac{T - m_1 g}{m_1} \quad m_2: a = \frac{m_2 g - T}{m_2}$$

Setting the expressions equal to each other and solving for T yields:

$$T = g \left(\frac{2 m_1 m_2}{m_1 + m_2}\right)$$

Substituting all given information yields the tension, T:

$$T = \left(9.8 \frac{m}{s^2}\right) \left(\frac{2 \cdot 0.11 \text{ kg} \cdot 0.19 \text{ kg}}{0.11 \text{ kg} + 0.19 \text{ kg}}\right) = 1.37 \text{ N} \approx 1.4 \text{ N}$$

41. **The correct answer is A.** To find the effect of pulley friction on the system in Atwood's machine, one must first apply Newton's second law to the system:

$$\sum F_{net} = m_2 g - m_1 g - f = (m_1 + m_2) \, a$$

where downward is considered to be positive. Solving for the acceleration yields:

$$a = \frac{m_2 g - m_1 g - f}{(m_1 + m_2)}$$

42. **The correct answer is D.** This question requires basic knowledge of the equation of a line which is:

$$y = mx + b$$

where y is the y variable, x is the x variable, m is the slope, and b is the y intercept. The acceleration of the system using a pulley with friction is:

$$a = \frac{m_2 g - m_1 g - f}{(m_1 + m_2)}$$

which can be rewritten as:

$$a = \frac{(m_2 - m_1) \, g}{(m_1 + m_2)} - \frac{f}{(m_1 + m_2)}$$

$$= \frac{g}{(m_1 + m_2)} (m_2 - m_1) - \frac{f}{(m_1 + m_2)}$$

where a is the y-variable, $\dfrac{g}{(m_1 + m_2)}$ is the slope (m), ($m_2 - m_1$) is the x-variable, and $\dfrac{-f}{(m_1 + m_2)}$ is the y-intercept. Calculating the y-intercept from the graph and substituting for the two masses, one can calculate the frictional force, given by choice D.

43. **The correct answer is C.** The chromate esters of their hydrates cannot decompose by proton loss. Both ketones and aldehydes form carbonyl hydrates, and those hydrates form equilibrium quantities of chromate ester. However, in the case of ketones, the decomposition of the inorganic ester would require the departure of a carbocation, for which there is a considerably higher barrier than for a proton.

44. **The correct answer is B.** Without water, no carbonyl hydrate can be formed, thus trapping the aldehyde at that stage.

45. **The correct answer is D.** The most likely product would be an oxo aldehyde. Jones conditions will oxidize the secondary alcohol to the ketone and the primary alcohol to the carboxylic acid.

46. **The correct answer is C.** The most likely product would be an oxo aldehyde. The PCC will oxidize the secondary alcohol to the ketone and the primary alcohol to the aldehyde.

47. **The correct answer is A.** The most likely compound isolated is an alcohol. For much the same reason that ketones do not overoxidize, tertiary alcohols are resistant to oxidation by chromium (VI) reagents, since it would require the departure of a carbocation in the chromate ester decomposition step.

48. **The correct answer is B.** α-D-Glucose and β-D-glucose differ by a single stereocenter. If one or more—but not all—stereocenters are different, the two compounds are diastereomers. In an enantiomer, each and every stereocenter must have changed. Thus, the enantiomer of D-glucose is L-glucose:

49. **The correct answer is A.** The hemiacetal functionality is highlighted in glucose shown. Note that the hemiacetal carbon is in the same oxidation state as a carbonyl group, which is revealed by two bonds to oxygen. In an acetal, two alkoxy groups are attached to one carbon; in a hemiacetal, one is a hydroxy group and the other is an alkoxy group:

50. **The correct answer is B.** Mutarotation involves the cleavage of the hemiacetal to form an intermediate aldehyde, which can reform the hemiacetal with different stereochemistry:

51. **The correct answer is C.** The difference between hexoses and pentoses is in the total number of carbons contained in the sugar—hexoses are C6 compounds and pentoses are C5 compounds. The difference between furanoses and pyranoses is in the size of the ring formed—furanoses form 5-membered rings and pyranoses form 6-membered rings. The nomenclature is derived from the simple cyclic ethers:

furan   pyran

52. **The correct answer is A.** With respect to the lone pairs on the ring oxygen, the β-hydroxy group suffers from unfavorable dipole-dipole interactions, whereas the α-isomer minimizes this electrostatic repulsion, resulting in lower energy:

53. **The correct answer is C.** All nitrates and chlorides are soluble. However, chlorides of silver, lead, and mercury are not soluble. The expected product is silver chloride.

54. **The correct answer is C.** At 100°C, the amount of NaCl dissolved will be 39.12 grams. But because this amount is per 100 mL of water, you need to adjust for using 250 mL of water. Doing so, you get 39.12 grams × 2.5 = 97.8 grams dissolving in 250 mL of water. At 0°C, the saturated solution will hold 35.7 grams × 2.5 = 89.3 grams. So the difference of 8.6 grams will precipitate out of solution.

55. **The correct answer is C.** In order to conduct electricity, there must be free ions in solution. By creating products that are insoluble, the number of free ions is minimal.

56. **The correct answer is A.** All sodium salts are soluble. Looking over the other choices, there are compounds containing other cations that are sometimes soluble and sometimes not. The experimental data indicate that the only true statement here is choice A.

57. **The correct answer is D.** The first three choices are all false statements. Silver nitrate is an example of a soluble silver compound. Sodium phosphate is an example of a soluble phosphate compound. An example of a soluble sulfate compound is ammonium sulfate. Looking at choice D, you have the following reaction in water: $AgCl(s) \longleftrightarrow Ag^+ (aq) + Cl^- (aq)$. The addition of ammonia to the solution forms a complex ion with silver ion. This reaction proceeds as: $Ag^+ (aq) + 2NH_3 (aq) \rightarrow Ag(NH_3)_2^+ (aq)$. As the ammonia removes the silver ions from solution, the equilibrium is shifted to the right and the silver chloride becomes more soluble.

58. **The correct answer is B.** Looking at the choices, three of the pairs are conjugate acid-base pairs, which differ by an H^+. However, choice B has the two substances differing by two H^+ ions. The conjugate base of sulfuric acid would be HSO_4^-. HSO_4^- would also be the conjugate acid of SO_4^{2-}.

59. **The correct answer is D.** Choice D shows all correct charges and coefficients for the equation. Five moles of calcium ions contribute $+10$. Three moles of phosphate ions contribute -9. One mole of hydroxide ions contributes -1. Adding them together results in a net of zero, signifying that the overall charge of the products is equal to the charge of the reactant.

60. **The correct answer is A.** The direction will lie toward the species that is the stronger base. Because hydroxide is a stronger base than fluoride, the equilibrium will lie to the right.

61. **The correct answer is B.** A larger K_{sp} means that the substance is more soluble and that more ions will be produced. Because the ions are the products, a larger K_{sp} means that the products predominate.

62. **The correct answer is B.** A common ion lowers the solubility of the salt. An increase in calcium ion is an increase in the concentration of a product. The equilibrium will then shift to the left so as to consume this increase and make more reactant.

63. **The correct answer is D.** Choice D shows the correct Lewis structure for fluoride ion. Fluorine atom starts with seven valence electrons. Adding one more electron to complete the octet, produces an ion with a negative one charge.

64. **The correct answer is D.** A total of nine ions are formed when hydroxyapatite dissolves. Because the coefficient of each ion becomes the power of the concentration, you have $[x]^5 \cdot [x]^3 \cdot [x]^1 = [x]^9$.

65. **The correct answer is D.** The first step of this problem is to convert the pressure in units of mmHg to pressure in units of N/m^2 using the given conversion factor:

$$P = 120\,\text{mmHg} \times \left(\frac{1333\,\frac{N}{m^2}}{1\,\text{mmHg}} \right) = 1.6 \times 10^5\,\frac{N}{m^2}$$

The second step is to determine the cross-sectional area of the aorta:

$$A = \pi r^2 = \pi \left(\frac{d}{2} \right)^2 = (3.14)\left(\frac{0.03\,m}{2} \right)^2 = 7.1 \times 10^{-4}\,m^2$$

Force is related to pressure and area by:

$$\text{Force} = \text{Pressure} \times \text{Area} = \left(1.6 \times 10^5\,\frac{N}{m^2} \right) \times (7.1 \times 10^{-4}\,m^2) = 114\,N$$

Section 3. Psychological, Social, and Biological Foundations of Behavior

1. **The correct answer is C.** Alfred cannot use retinal disparity because one of his eyes is closed. Retinal disparity occurs when the brain processes the difference in the images each eye receives and, using each visual perspective, integrates them into a 3-D representation of the environment.

2. **The correct answer is A.** Conflict theory states that society is fundamentally in conflict when there is an uneven distribution of resources, and that power struggles between groups of people create divisiveness across gender, race, and socioeconomic status.

3. **The correct answer is A.** The bystander effect is characterized by slowness in response due to diffusion of responsibility. The more people who are present, the less an individual is likely to feel responsible to respond to the emergency because of the collective presence of other individuals.

4. **The correct answer is A.** Functionalism sees aspects of society as separate but interrelated. Society as a whole is likened to a human body, in which each component acts separately but is critical to the functioning as a whole. In this view, a disruption to one area can disrupt the entire system. This view supports the status quo and attempts to avoid any disruptions to the system.

5. **The correct answer is C.** Altruism is more likely to occur between individuals who are likely to reciprocate assistance in the future. Studies of altruistic behavior have shown that helping others occurs more frequently among family members and in smaller communities and where it is most likely to be reciprocated in the future.

6. **The correct answer is B.** During variable-ratio trials the rat is reinforced after a specific number of bar presses. The number of presses varies over time. As a result, the rat presses the bar more vigorously. Further, this type of reinforcement has a higher resistance to extinction because the reinforcement schedule itself varies.

7. **The correct answer is C.** Conditioning would occur more slowly, and the slope in each cell would be flatter. The longer the delay between the response and reinforcement, the more slowly conditioning occurs.

8. **The correct answer is D.** Fixed-ratio responses are characterized by a high rate of bar presses, and the short break taken by the rat is indicative of a fixed period of bar presses. Under fixed reinforcement the rat will press the bar quickly because responses are tied to the number of presses and not a time interval.

9. **The correct answer is C.** Ratio reinforcement usually results in predictable response patterns under each of the conditions (fixed and variable), with steady responding in a 1:1 ratio, and multiple rapid bar presses in the variable response ratio condition with long breaks in between. The variable nature of the reinforcement results in greater resistance to extinction in later trials as the rat continues

with the behavior even in the absence of reinforcement in hopes of eventually getting a reinforcement.

10. **The correct answer is A.** In operant conditioning the stimulus always precedes the reinforcement or punishment. In the model of operant conditioning, the punishment or reinforcement of a behavior results in the increase or decrease of that behavior. The behavior is elicited by the stimulus and therefore precedes the conditioning.

11. **The correct answer is A.** The largest proportion of responders are in the conventional level because most people never reach the postconventional level. This is consistent with Kohlberg's model and is expected based on the data pattern.

12. **The correct answer is C.** Conventional morality develops between the ages of 7 and 16. It develops as preconventional morality extinguishes. The key period for this change is between 7 and 16 years old.

13. **The correct answer is B.** Moral judgments can be understood in context based on stages of moral development. In Kohlberg's model, the reasons given by the research subjects for answering questions a particular way defined which level of development was being exhibited.

14. **The correct answer is D.** Stage 3 morality is characterized by the basing of decisions on personally constructed moral principles rather than on the likelihood of reward or punishment, or society's rules or laws. According to Kohlberg, someone functioning at this level would be able to reject personal fulfillment and unjust laws in order to make moral decisions.

15. **The correct answer is B.** James is displaying behavior consistent with the conventional stage of moral development. In this stage decisions are based on society's rules and laws with judgments based on relatively absolute criteria (black/white, right/wrong).

16. **The correct answer is B.** Changing the location of the comparison light allows researchers to isolate where the light from the test stimuli reaches the retina. When the comparison light is located at the fixation point, the light falls on the fovea, where the cones are located. When the test light is presented away from the fixation point (in the periphery), the rods are activated.

17. **The correct answer is A.** The participant is considered to have detected the light if he or she can identify the comparison light presence 50% of the time. Using signal detection, the presence and absence of the test light is manipulated along with the intensity of the light.

18. **The correct answer is D.** The rods are maximally sensitive after 20 minutes in the dark and are more sensitive overall. Cones are initially more sensitive than rods but become less so after the rod-cone break. At the breakpoint, cones and rods are equally sensitive. Rods only become more sensitive at a lower level of light after the breakpoint.

19. **The correct answer is C.** Rods cannot distinguish between different wavelengths, therefore rod-based light perception is on the black and white gradient and is the primary form of human visual perception after the rod-cone break.

20. **The correct answer is D.** Rods are better at light adaptation because large groups of them are connected to one interneuron. The interneuron amplifies the signal from each rod receptor decreasing resolution while increasing overall sensitivity to light.

21. **The correct answer is D.** The individual spent a longer amount of time solving algebra problems in a group compared to solving them alone.

22. **The correct answer is B.** The results are consistent with social loafing. This concept is exemplified when an individual reduces his or her effort on a task based on the assumption that other members of the group will "step up" to complete the task.

23. **The correct answer is A.** Social facilitation is exemplified when an individual increases his or her effort on a task in a group situation; completing it faster and more accurately.

24. **The correct answer is B.** The individual would reduce the amount of effort spent on solving the problems because he or she would assume others would step up to complete the task. This result is consistent with social loafing, which posits that as group size and task complexity increase, the amount of effort expended by individuals decreases.

25. **The correct answer is A.** The effort expended is the result of the participant's perception of diffusion of responsibility. Social loafing is characterized by the reduction in effort by individuals when they work in groups. This result is consistent even when individuals *think* that they are working alone regardless of whether or not they are *actually* working alone. The individual's perception about the presence of others is more critical to this process than the actuality of the presence of others.

26. **The correct answer is A.** Men in the United States rated physical attractiveness at the highest level across cultures.

27. **The correct answer is C.** The similarity in results shows that mate selection preferences are universal and likely due to evolutionary influences. Learning varies across cultures, so mate selection preferences are unlikely to be wholly learned.

28. **The correct answer is B.** Women focus more on financial status than men do when selecting mates because they are driven to maximize the material resources that can be invested in children. This answer is consistent with evolutionary psychology, which characterizes human behavior in terms of evolutionary drives and seeks to identify behaviors that are true across cultures, which may be due to adaptive evolutionary pressures.

29. **The correct answer is C.** A useful follow-up study would ask participants located in an extremely remote society to complete the same survey used in this example.

Asking participants from an extremely remote society may help to further determine whether the characteristics are universal.

30. **The correct answer is A.** Evolutionary psychology suggests that human behavior evolved due to natural selection. It posits that human behavior was shaped by characteristics of the environment through natural selection, resulting in the behavior humans exhibit today. Evolutionary psychologists often look for measurements that remain constant regardless of cultural variations as candidates for study.

31. **The correct answer is C.** Individuals identifying as "African American" are more likely to be diagnosed with schizophrenia, and individuals who identify as "White" are more likely to be diagnosed with a mood disorder.

32. **The correct answer is C.** Clinicians see no ethnicity differences in admittance rates for some disorders. This conclusion can be ruled out because the observable data collected contradict this statement. However, it is not possible to determine the degree of influence that ethnicity has on the rates of diagnoses or on the incidence rate in these studies since it only assesses those admitted for psychiatric care. It does not measure the rate of diagnosis or population prevalence of psychiatric disorders.

33. **The correct answer is A.** A logical follow-up study would measure the social and economic status and stress of each person diagnosed with schizophrenia and mood disorder. This is the most correct answer because such a study would further investigate the environmental causes for mental disorders. This additional research also fits with the vulnerability-stress view of schizophrenia.

34. **The correct answer is D.** A person has a 100% chance of developing schizophrenia if both of his or her parents have schizophrenia. This answer is incorrect because even though schizophrenia is heritable, genetic factors alone are not responsible for the development of the disorder and a child inherits 50% of each parent's genotype. This would not guarantee that a child would receive the genetic sequence that is required to be susceptible to this complex, polygenic disorder of schizophrenia.

35. **The correct answer is A.** The more stress to which a person who is genetically predisposed to schizophrenia is exposed, the greater the likelihood that person will experience a psychotic break. The vulnerability-stress view suggests that environmental stressors are correlated to the expression of schizophrenic symptoms. As these stressors increase, the likelihood increases that a person biologically predisposed to schizophrenia will exhibit symptoms. The research is still ongoing with regard to answer C and the vulnerability-stress model does not currently recognize differences in positive and negative stress. Answer D would require the individual to experience stress along with the biological family to fulfill the requirements of the model. If the individual was adopted and has no contact with the biological family, the biological family's stress will not trigger a schizophrenic break.

36. **The correct answer is C.** Commitment initially increases slowly; then it rapidly increases. The model depicts commitment increasing slowly. Then as passion begins to drop, commitment increases rapidly.

37. **The correct answer is C.** Commitment is crucial and is positively correlated to relationship stability. Various studies have shown that commitment is predictive of relationship stability. Commitment is also shown in the model to be at the highest level for the greatest length of time.

38. **The correct answer is A.** Romantic love is characterized by intense emotions and sexual feelings. The passion component develops quickly and early in the relationship and declines rapidly as commitment increases.

39. **The correct answer is D.** Companionate love develops over time and is characterized in Sternberg's model by commitment and intimacy. Choice A is incorrect because if the individual components that make up fatuous love and liking were present, it would be consummate love.

40. **The correct answer is D.** Although Danna has been with Mark for some time, their relationship is best categorized as infatuation due to the lack of commitment and intimacy in the context of strong sexual feelings.

41. **The correct answer is B.** The majority of state average scores were above the national average. Sixteen of the states listed were below the national average and 34 were above. Most state average scores exceeded the national average.

42. **The correct answer is D.** Conflict theory posits that the difference in prestige and resources creates fundamental power struggles between groups of people and that these power struggles create divisiveness across groups. In the example given, the sociologist is examining differences in groups that are historically underperforming and evaluating how power divisiveness is being minimized.

43. **The correct answer is C.** The data reflect attempts to reinforce the status quo between various state populations. Functionalists view education as structured in such a way that it reinforces the status quo. It keeps societies stable and seeks to avoid disruptions in the system.

44. **The correct answer is C.** Teaching in the state school system is part of the service, or tertiary, sector of the economy. The primary sector includes the extractive industries such as mining and forestry. The secondary sector includes the manufacturing industries.

45. **The correct answer is B.** Jim is attempting to maintain the status quo and is attempting to prevent disruptions in the existing system. His work is consistent with functionalism.

46. **The correct answer is D.** The share of the elderly population in Japan will increase over time relative to the rest of the population. In the graphs, the share of elderly people, shown as the top portion of each population "pyramid," is projected to increase over time relative to the shares of young and adult persons (shown as the bottom and middle portions of each population "pyramid").

47. **The correct answer is B.** There would be fewer transitional youth in the population in 2060 than in 2020. The transitional youth category is an additional age group between the ages of 15 and 30. It would overlap the existing youth and adult populations and would show the same overall pattern of reduction shown in both those populations over time.

48. **The correct answer is A.** Social and cultural characteristics would become more diverse across the population. This result is consistent with more mobile societies and reflects the changing demographics that would be evident from an addition of individuals from different backgrounds.

49. **The correct answer is B.** The elderly are likely to have more influence on public policy as their share of the population increases.

50. **The correct answer is D.** The ethnicity of the overall population would remain basically the same. Ethnicity is a social construct, and if the immigrants became culturally integrated into the native culture, that would not change the ethnicity of the overall population. Race, on the other hand, is determined by biological and genetic factors. Racial composition may or may not change with an immigrant group, depending on the biological makeup of the original and immigrant groups.

51. **The correct answer is B.** Latino individuals are as likely as white individuals to have access to minimally adequate mental health treatment post diagnosis. While Latino individuals are less likely than whites to be diagnosed with mental illness, they are as likely to receive minimally adequate treatment post diagnosis.

52. **The correct answer is B.** Individuals of lower socioeconomic status (SES) who have mental health difficulties have fewer financial resources and less access to mental health care, and are therefore less able to seek treatment. The culture of poverty theory would ignore the reduced access to mental health treatment and attribute George's problems to his poor choices related to drug use. This scenario speaks against social mobility rather than describes it. Human capital does not apply because George has the education to improve his SES.

53. **The correct answer is B.** As a young person with no financial resources, George has less access to mental health care. Additionally, now that he is no longer a student, he likely does not have access to the student counseling center at his school.

54. **The correct answer is C.** Both the stigma related to seeking mental health care and the lack of mental health providers in lower SES areas are likely to affect George's ability to receive treatment.

55. **The correct answer is A.** While black individuals are the least likely to receive a mental health diagnosis, they also have the least access to minimally adequate mental health treatment and are the least likely to receive treatment once diagnosed.

56. **The correct answer is A.** Bodily resources are mobilized and metabolism speeds up. During the alarm stage people experience increased physiological arousal. They will become anxious and frightened. The response is similar to the fight-or-flight syndrome.

57. **The correct answer is D.** Resistance; the reaction can persist for hours, days, or years. In GAS, people experiencing resistance generally have a negative emotional and physical reaction (e.g., being tired, irritable, impatient, and angry). However, they are able to intentionally engage in adaptive stress management activities (meditation, seeking social support) to reduce the negative impact of stress. Exhaustion is characterized by extreme physical and mental fatigue. However, it is also characterized by the lack of ability to engage in adaptive stress management activities to resist stress.

58. **The correct answer is B.** Resistance reactions are adaptive and can help reduce the impact of stress. This is consistent with GAS theory. Resistance reactions are those activities that the individual uses to resist the negative impact of stress on the mind and body in order to reduce the likelihood of entering the exhaustion stage.

59. **The correct answer is B.** Multiple simultaneous stressors may overwhelm an individual's stress resistance activities and push him or her into the exhaustion stage more quickly. Individuals are able to resist stress until it overwhelms their adaptive resistance activities, after which the individual falls into exhaustion. Multiple simultaneous moderately stressful events will impact the efficacy of stress resistance activities and push the individual into the exhaustion stage faster than only a single stressor of moderate severity.

60. **The correct answer is A.** Jeremy reacted by adapting and making behavioral changes in response to the stressful situation in an attempt to reduce the stress. This is a characteristic of a resistance reaction.

61. **The correct answer is C.** The forgetting curve is characterized by an initial rapid decrease in the proportion remembered, followed by a slow flattening out over time.

62. **The correct answer is D.** Based on the forgetting curve, each relearning episode increases the amount retained over time. Recall is better for the first few days with each relearning episode.

63. **The correct answer is D.** Relearning impacts the rate of forgetting only after several relearning episodes. In the graph, relearning impacts the rate of forgetting as early as the first relearning episode, although repeated relearning episodes slow the rate of forgetting. Even in the context of multiple relearning episodes, forgetting does still occur over time, but repetition slows this rate of loss.

64. **The correct answer is A.** Test performance would decline sharply at first but decline less and less in later years. There is no relearning in this scenario and the results would be consistent with the slope of the forgetting curve.

65. **The correct answer is D.** There would be a significant decline in your memory in the first week, but the decline would become less abrupt after each time that you studied the list. Each relearning interval will increase the amount retained on subsequent tests.

Section 4. Critical Analysis and Reasoning Skills

1. **The correct answer is D.** The woolly flying squirrel did not really vanish; *salajit* collectors knew of its existence. Choices A, B, and C are supported by information in the passage.

2. **The correct answer is C.** Zahler chooses not to track the aquatic genet because he prefers to look for a creature that does not live in a tropical biome. There is no support for the notion that tropical diseases affect these mammals (choice D). The other two choices may or may not be true, but they are not supported by the author's mention of the genet in the article.

3. **The correct answer is D.** Paragraph 1 gives MacKinnon's requirements for rediscovery or discovery of species. The woolly flying squirrel's home in caves in the Himalayas certainly meets the requirement for isolation (choice A), but as paragraph 4 points out, it also meets the requirements for geographic and climatic stability, making choice D the correct answer.

4. **The correct answer is B.** The discussion of how Zahler chose this animal to study appears in paragraph 3. He wanted a mammal that was not too small, relatively unknown, and in need of conservation intervention. Because he did not wish to deal with heat or diseases, he passed up the aquatic genet for the woolly flying squirrel. That makes choice B the best answer.

5. **The correct answer is A.** To answer this question, you must apply MacKinnon's requirements to your knowledge of geography. MacKinnon suggests that dry climates are not conducive to rediscovery, making the Sahara an unlikely answer (choice D). Western Iran is prone to earthquake activity, making it a less likely choice than the more remote, steamy jungles of Borneo. Choice A is the best answer.

6. **The correct answer is A.** Information that weakens the argument will argue against rediscovery's being a way to protect species. Of the information given, choices B, C, and D suggest ways that species are being protected. Only choice A mentions something that might actually harm a rediscovered species.

7. **The correct answer is D.** Both the Beat and the Lost Generations came of age during war and found it hard to cope in the postwar world. Both tended toward exile and alienation, making choice D the best answer.

8. **The correct answer is C.** The word *culture* is used twice—to refer to "the drug culture" and to "sixties culture." Choices A, B, and D make no sense in this context, so the only possible connotation is choice C.

9. **The correct answer is B.** According to the author, "the trials loosened some of the definitions that had bound American literature." The trials, then, did not affect the movement of the Beats (choice A) or their influences (choice C); they affected modern definitions of literature (choice B).

10. **The correct answer is B.** To answer this question correctly, you must ask yourself, "Is there at least one example of I, II, or III anywhere in the passage?" Statement I

says that Kerouac continued to write before his *On the Road* was published, but there are no examples of what he wrote. Statement III says that the Beats influenced sixties culture, but there are no examples of works from that era that showed the Beats' influence. Statement II says that the drug culture affected some Beats. The author gives the example of Burroughs, who wrote *Junkie* about his own addiction, and also mentions "Howl" and its emphasis on drug culture. Because only statement II has supporting examples, the only correct response is (choice B).

11. **The correct answer is C.** It is the subject matter, not the form of Corso's poetry that ties it to the angst of a postwar generation. Including "Bomb" in the passage would help support the point made in choice C.

12. **The correct answer is D.** If the Beats were omitted from an important anthology, it could only indicate that they were not considered important enough to include. That would negate choice D, the notion that they transcended their time. It would not say anything about choice A or C, and the fact that Beat writing was difficult (choice B) would not be enough to eliminate it from an anthology.

13. **The correct answer is C.** Refining is one of the three steps in the creation of aluminum. It involves the separation of a solution through distillation and addition of chemicals. Although *refined* is a multiple-meaning word that in context may have any of the four definitions listed, only choice C works in the context of this passage.

14. **The correct answer is B.** Choice A is true, but it has nothing to do with the protests. There is no evidence to support choice D. Choice C may or may not be true; it is implied, but it is not a major point. The mention of protests mainly indicates choice B, that workers are beginning to question the dangers of mining.

15. **The correct answer is A.** There is nothing to support choice B or C, and the author is completely objective when it comes to the discussion of Karl Bayer (choice D). In the final paragraph, the author states, "As with all mining of metals, bauxite mining presents certain hazards," indicating that choice A is the best answer.

16. **The correct answer is C.** Paragraph 6 describes the process of refinement and its by-products. Those that are mentioned in the paragraph include choices A, B, and D. There is no mention of choice C, which is an alloy of aluminum and an element not involved in this refining process.

17. **The correct answer is D.** According to paragraph 2, the most commonly mined form of bauxite is gibbsite, a trihydrate form of bauxite. If it is trihydrate, then it contains three molecules of water (choice D). There is no evidence in the passage to support any of the other choices.

18. **The correct answer is B.** The three-step process that produces aluminum is described as involving mining, refining, and smelting. It is typical of the process that results in most metal products that we use, so it is parallel to copper production (choice B). None of the other three products results from the same three-step process.

19. **The correct answer is C.** The final paragraph mentions Bowdler's works other than Shakespeare and discusses the fact that we derive a verb from his name. The main idea of the paragraph, however, is that Bowdler's form of editing continues to the present day (choice C); several examples of present-day bowdlerization are given.

20. **The correct answer is B.** Bowdler himself was trained as a doctor; the passage makes clear that he was not an editor. His sister, however, was a poet and editor, and therefore was more likely than he to have made the editorial changes that led to the revised Shakespearean texts. There is no evidence in the passage to support choice C or D, and although there is some implication that choice A is true, it does not explain why she would have been a more likely editor than he.

21. **The correct answer is A.** There is no mention of a dream (choice D), the poet laureate is used as an example of prior editing but not as an inspiration for Bowdler himself (choice C), and Bowdler was not a scholar, making choice B an unlikely answer. Instead, his desire was to make Shakespeare accessible to children, and in its unexpurgated state, he felt that was impossible. Choice A is the best answer.

22. **The correct answer is D.** Look for the answer that is supported by the text. Although choices A, B, and C may in fact be true, none of them receives support in the passage. The author's reason for including mention of Nehum Tate is to show that the Bowdlers were not the first to edit Shakespeare.

23. **The correct answer is C.** Remember that the answer will NOT be an example of bowdlerization. First, you must find the definition of bowdlerization in the text: "to censor or amend a written work, often with a connotation of prudishness." Item I is not an example of this; simply translating from one language to another requires neither censorship or amendment. Item III is not an example either; although some may say that book burning is a radical form of censorship, it does not fit the definition here. Only II, which deals with the censorship of a detail in a text, fits the definition. Since I and III do not, choice C is the correct answer.

24. **The correct answer is A.** Although choices B, C, and D appear in the passage, none of them supports the claim that Bowdler's revised Shakespeare was not universally despised. The quote from Swinburne (choice A), however, does—Swinburne praises Bowdler for creating a Shakespeare that can be put in the hands of children.

25. **The correct answer is A.** Because the author makes the point that bowdlerization still occurs today, it is not likely that everyone would revile such a text (choice B) or see that it failed (choice D). More likely would be that it would receive some condemnation but also make some sales (choice A). Although a point is made about "dumbing down" texts for high school students (choice C), the author does not appear to support this, nor is it proof that students would not understand the bowdlerized Shakespeare.

26. **The correct answer is B.** "The Red Cross, yes, but Henry Kissinger?" asks the author. The author finds the controversy over Rigoberta "surprising" and states,

"her place in the history of Central American peasant revolutions seems assured." That indicates that as far as the author is concerned, the committee's choice of Rigoberta is not undeserved (I), but the choice of Kissinger may well be (II). Since the author gives the Red Cross (III) a thumbs-up, only choice B fits the passage.

27. **The correct answer is C.** For vocabulary-in-context questions like this one, always locate the word in question because the distracters are likely to be alternate meanings of that word. Here, the passage states, "Rigoberta's father was taken into custody and tortured when the army believed he had assisted in the assassination of a plantation owner." The only answer that makes sense in this context is choice C.

28. **The correct answer is C.** The question asks you to find the one or more statements that do NOT support the premise that Rigoberta falsified her book. To do that, you must find the statements that do support that premise and eliminate those. Statements that do support the premise will indicate some kind of disconnect between what she said and what was true. Those statements include I and II. Statement III, on the other hand, is simply a statement of fact. It does not support the premise that she falsified the book. The answer is choice C.

29. **The correct answer is B.** This question calls for a cause-and-effect relationship. You must find the cause of Rigoberta's departure. That is not simply something that happened before her departure (choice D), or something that was true but not a direct cause (choice A). The cause appears in the sentence "Soon Rigoberta was herself a target." She left because otherwise she might have been assassinated (choice B).

30. **The correct answer is D.** This question is purely speculative, since the author did not include information to support the statement. If the author had, it would have had to be information that told more about the teaching of Rigoberta's book in schools. Two students' comments (choice A) would not be enough evidence, and choices B and C might show that the book is still sold but not that it is widely taught. Only choice D includes reasonable evidence.

31. **The correct answer is C.** You are asked here to assess the relative relevance of evidence. Falsifying a birth date (choice A) might be evidence of a minor deception, but it would not be enough to support charges of fraud. Falsifying a critical part of her history as it relates to her reputation, as choice C would do, would certainly indicate a desire to deceive.

32. **The correct answer is A.** David Stoll objects to what he considers Rigoberta's misleading the public on matters of fact. That would not mean that her work was an epic (choice B) or a folktale (choice C) because those are specific genres of literature that do not fit his accusations. Nor would he call her work a manifesto (choice D) because he does not accept her as a leader. He might, however, use the trendy word *truthiness* to describe what he feels to be a bending of the truth.

33. **The correct answer is C.** To answer this kind of question, you must compare what you know about the author's point of view with the choices given. The author, unlike some of the people in the passage, seems to have a positive view of Rigoberta, as evinced in the line, "her place in the history of Central American peasant revolutions seems assured." That means that choices A and B would be unlikely views of this author, and there is no evidence to support choice D one way or the other. The best answer is choice C.

34. **The correct answer is D.** The author finds that metanarratives are often racist, sexist, or classist; but that mininarratives are often too restrictive or exclusive to be useful. The best answer is choice D.

35. **The correct answer is C.** You must make this prediction based on what the author has said in the passage. Two examples of courses in American history are given to support the notion that some mininarratives are incompatible, but there is no indication that offering more courses would help (choice A). The author mentions revising the canon (choice B) in paragraphs 4 and 5 but implies that it was a good and necessary idea. Red states and blue states are mentioned in passing, but there is little else to indicate the author's feelings about politics (choice D). The best answer is choice C; the author is concerned that students today find it hard to see a "big picture" due to their immersion in competing mininarratives.

36. **The correct answer is D.** Supposition I is supported by the examples of competing American history courses. Supposition II is supported by the clash between evolutionary theory and strict Bible interpretation. Supposition III is supported by the example of a Eurocentric look at American history (see paragraph 2). Since all three suppositions are supported by examples, choice D is the best answer.

37. **The correct answer is B.** The main idea of the passage has to do with the tension between metanarratives and mininarratives, especially as they affect the way we learn things. This would be most useful for people who develop curricula.

38. **The correct answer is B.** *Smorgasbord* is a Swedish word meaning "a buffet meal featuring a variety of dishes." It is this variety, or choice, to which the author refers. Even if you do not know the word, you should be able to guess this from context.

39. **The correct answer is D.** All three philosophies are all-encompassing ways to look at the world, so all three could be considered metanarratives. Since all three are valid, the answer is choice D.

40. **The correct answer is A.** A mininarrative looks at the world through a limited lens. A metanarrative provides more of a big picture. The best analogy is choice A.

41. **The correct answer is C.** This question asks you to find the main idea. To find the main idea, you must read actively and summarize as you go. There are no titles on MCAT passages to reveal the central thesis, so you must derive it from the text. To determine the correct answer, review the choices. You need to select the one that is not only true according to the passage, but also not so specific

that it excludes one or more of the author's main points. The author indicates that millions of people are blogging but does not mention how many people read popular blogs. Therefore choice A is not supported by the text and can be eliminated. Similarly, the author notes that advertisers are spending more money on blogs than they have in the past but does not reveal that traditional print and broadcasting outlets are receiving less money (choice B). While choice D is true according to the passage, it is not general enough to be the central thesis. Choice C is the correct response, echoing the general statement made at the beginning of the passage, and being broad enough to encompass the author's points made throughout the text.

42. **The correct answer is B.** This question asks you to draw conclusions about a fact presented in the passage. It is a skill most often applied to fiction, but it works in this case for nonfiction as well. The word *implies* tells you that the answer is not directly stated. It is up to you to return to the passage and make inferences based on what is written. The passage states that *popular* bloggers are the ones making money from advertising. There is no general information given about what makes a blog popular; one blogger earns money from humor, while another presents controversial political discourse. There is nothing in the passage to suggest that content about celebrities equates with popularity, eliminating choice C. There is also no reason given to infer that bloggers are, or should be, appealing to marketers (choice D). Although there is one example of a popular blog that is controversial, the other example regarding a humorous website makes choice B the correct answer. Marketers want to advertise on sites that are read by many people, regardless of content.

43. **The correct answer is A.** You must apply new evidence to an assertion in the passage for this question. Specifically, what fact presented by the author would be challenged by evidence that traditional media sources were successfully competing for blogs' advertising revenue? Choices B and D are true statements according to the passage, but they do not relate to the new evidence and should be eliminated. There is nothing in the passage to suggest that blogs are better at disseminating information, so choice C should also be eliminated. A careful rereading of the final paragraph reveals that marketers spend money on blogs and other online advertising because they want "new and more effective ways to reach consumers." Therefore, choice A is correct.

44. **The correct answer is C.** This question involves analyzing an argument. The assertion that blogs influence language (I) is supported by the example of a dictionary giving the distinction of "word of the year" to *blog*. There is no example given of politicians using blogs for any reason (II). Since the assertion that blogs include otherwise neglected news (III) is supported by the story about Trent Lott, both I and III are true, and choice C is correct.

45. **The correct answer is C.** This question tests your ability to locate supporting details or evidence. In questions of this kind, everything you need to know is found directly in the text. The last line of paragraph 2 contains the information: "When those passive consumers use simple websites to disseminate facts and ideas of their choosing, they evolve from passive consumers to active participants, effectively blurring the line between the media and its audience." There is nothing in the passage to suggest that the advertising revenue diverted to blogs is changing the nature of the media (choice A). While the passage does present evidence that blogs can affect political careers (choice B) and they are a public display of ideas (choice D), this evidence is not related to a change in the nature of the media. Choice C is the only correct response.

46. **The correct answer is D.** For questions such as this one, you must draw a conclusion by going beyond the facts of the passage to determine the correct answer. The coverage of Senator Lott is an example of the expansion of what is considered to be newsworthy, not an example of how blogs are attracting advertisers and their money (choice A). There is no suggestion that the coverage was designed to do anything other than report on the news, so choice B is also incorrect. Since Lott resigned from his position as Speaker of the House, the story was not ineffective, eliminating choice C. Choice D is the correct answer because paragraph 3 clearly states that traditional media sources often don't cover what they deem to be controversial news stories, "virtually ignoring" Lott's remarks.

47. **The correct answer is A.** This evaluation question asks you to analyze an argument. Specifically, you need to figure out why the author mentioned the Platonic tradition. In the first paragraph, the author states that the prevailing view of mathematics is an "easy" one that may be "cemented" in the minds of people. Later, in the third paragraph, the author states that the new view of mathematics has met with "stiff resistance." Thus, the mention of the Platonic tradition helps to explain why there is resistance to the conclusions of the new paradigm, which is what choice A says.

48. **The correct answer is C.** To answer this question, you must assess evidence. Since this is an EXCEPT question, you're looking for the choice that is not present in the passage. The passage does discuss experiments, choice A, in the section about violation of expectation tests. The part about the PhD in chemistry who suffered from acalculia is a case study (choice B). Finally, the author presents a comparison (choice D) when showing how animals and humans have similar abilities. That leaves choice C as the correct answer.

49. **The correct answer is D.** This question asks you to draw conclusions about an assertion that is not directly stated. The second paragraph states that mathematics is created by man, which implies that mathematical concepts are to some degree arbitrary. Choice A is contradicted by the passage in the final paragraph when the

author says that the acalculia patient "has no problem manipulating abstract algebraic operations." Choice B is not supported because the passage only mentions that *some* animals have mathematical abilities. Choice C is incorrect; infants at the age of a few months can perform simple calculations. At younger ages they can only differentiate between two and three items.

50. **The correct answer is C.** This question involves interpreting vocabulary. The word *curious* appears in the final passage. In that paragraph, the author discusses "anomalous" cases and describes the situation as "strange." This makes choice C, "odd," the best choice. There is no indication that the author thinks the fact is superb or excellent ("marvelous," choice A), of foreign origin ("exotic," choice B), or new ("novel," choice D).

51. **The correct answer is A.** In order to answer this question, you must be able to judge credibility. The author cites the violation of expectation experiment as support for the author's claim that mathematics is an innate part of human cognition. In order for these experiments to be credible, the author is assuming that the researchers can accurately determine that the infants are in fact surprised when the number of puppets changes. The only evidence for this is the direction and duration of the stares of the subjects. Accepting these results as evidence indicates the author believes outward signs accurately indicate inner emotional states; otherwise, the evidence would not support the argument.

52. **The correct answer is C.** This question requires you to find the main idea. The passage states that a longstanding view of mathematics as an objective reality is being challenged by new evidence in the fields of cognitive science and developmental psychology. This is what choice C expresses. Choice A is incorrect because the main idea of the passage does not concern Western philosophers. The passage does not claim that animals have the same mathematical abilities as humans do, making choice B wrong. Choice D is not supported by the passage at all.

53. **The correct answer is D.** This question asks you to apply new evidence. This question is very difficult because you must understand both the nature of the author's argument and the effect of new evidence on it. The passage argues that mathematical thinking is a product of the innate structures of the brain and mathematical "truths" are created by people. Finding a group of people that lacks mathematical ability might seem to refute the argument as choice A indicates, but upon closer examination it is not the best answer. The author does allow that certain changes in the brain may destroy the ability to perform mathematical operations. Thus, the community of math-deficient people may have a genetic mutation that prevents them from doing math. If so, it would not harm the author's argument. If, however, the group had no brain abnormalities and possessed no mathematical abilities, it would challenge the author's belief that mathematical thought is hardwired into the brain. Thus, choice D is the best answer.

54. **The correct answer is C.** This question asks you to find the main idea. This passage discusses the basic structure of language and specifically a feature of the English language, namely its paucity of verb forms. Choice C is the best summary of the passage. Choice A is not the main idea of the passage at all. Choice B is too strong. It is not stated that each and every language is unique. Choice D is wrong because the passage states the English language is able to convey a number of meanings even though its verb forms are limited.

55. **The correct answer is A.** This application question asks you to draw conclusions. The author states that the English language makes do with fewer verb forms than other languages, but it still can convey different meanings. This makes choice A correct. Choices B and D are not supported by the passage, while choice C reflects what some linguists believe.

56. **The correct answer is C.** This question involves analyzing an argument. Statement I is supported by the examples of the Spanish language and the Kivunjo language, which have far more forms than the English language. Statement II is unsupported by a specific example. Statement III is supported by the example in the final paragraph of the different meanings of similar-sounding verb forms, which makes choice C the best answer.

57. **The correct answer is B.** In order to answer this question, you'll need to combine information. The passage provides interesting information on language and specifically on the English language. However, it is not directed at linguists (choice A), who presumably would already know much of the information. A language teacher (choice B) would most likely find the information interesting background to a language lesson. It is not clear what psychologists would find interesting in the passage. Translators may find the information interesting, but nothing in the passage pertains specifically to translation, so choice B is a better answer.

58. **The correct answer is B.** This question tests your ability to make predictions. Based on the information in the passage, you need to predict which sentence may strike a Spanish speaker as odd. The passage states that in Spanish, the stem of the verb is not a word. In English, one use of the stem of the verb is in the infinitive form, as used in choice B, "to see." The past tense (choice A), the third-person singular (choice C), and the gerund form (choice D) all involve changing the stem, which is similar to the Spanish language.

59. **The correct answer is B.** This question asks about supporting details. The passage states that the present tense (statement I) is usually expressed using the stem form of the verb but can also be expressed in the third-person singular by using the $-s$ suffix. Similarly, verbal adjectives (statement II) are sometimes expressed using the –*ing* suffix and sometimes with the –*ed* suffix.

60. **The correct answer is B.** This question requires you to draw conclusions. From the information in the passage, what can be concluded about the Russian language? Its lack of pronounceable stems for its verbs makes it similar to Spanish and different from English. Furthermore, the passage states that English is unlike many Indo-European languages in its use of the stem form as a word. From this information, a linguist may conclude that Russian might (but not necessarily) be part of the Indo-European family. Just because the stem forms are not pronounced gives no information on the number of forms as choice A states. Choice C is not a valid inference based on the information in the passage. The lack of pronounced stem verbs says nothing about the number of inflections, which are the ways a word changes when taking on different roles in the sentence.

EVALUATION CHART

Use this Evaluation Chart to analyze your results on the science sections (Sections 1, 2, and 3) of Practice Test 1. Check the Answers and Explanations section to see which answers you got correct and which ones you missed. For each question that you missed, find the question number in the left column of the chart below. Look in the right column to see the chapter in a companion volume in the **McGraw-Hill Education MCAT Test Preparation series** that covers the content area for that question. If you missed questions in a specific content area, you need to pay particular attention to that area as you study for the MCAT.

Item Number	Content Area
Biological and Biochemical Foundations of Living Systems	
	Chapter in *McGraw-Hill Education: MCAT Biological and Biochemical Foundations of Living Systems*
1.	Chapter 9: Structure and Integrative Functions of the Main Organ Systems
2.	Chapter 8: Structure and Function of the Nervous and Endocrine Systems and Ways in Which These Systems Coordinate the Organ Systems
3.	Chapter 2: Transmission of Genetic Information from the Gene to the Protein
4.	Chapter 6: Structure, Growth, Physiology, and Genetics of Prokaryotes and Viruses
5.	Chapter 3: Transmission of Heritable Information from Generation to Generation and the Processes That Increase Genetic Diversity
6.	Chapter 9: Structure and Integrative Functions of the Main Organ Systems
7.	Chapter 5: Assemblies of Molecules, Cells, and Groups of Cells Within Multicellular Organisms
8.	Chapter 9: Structure and Integrative Functions of the Main Organ Systems
9.	Chapter 5: Assemblies of Molecules, Cells, and Groups of Cells Within Multicellular Organisms
10.	Chapter 9: Structure and Integrative Functions of the Main Organ Systems
11.	Chapter 9: Structure and Integrative Functions of the Main Organ Systems
12.	Chapter 8: Structure and Function of the Nervous and Endocrine Systems and Ways in Which These Systems Coordinate the Organ Systems
13.	Chapter 9: Structure and Integrative Functions of the Main Organ Systems
14.	Chapter 8: Structure and Function of the Nervous and Endocrine Systems and Ways in Which These Systems Coordinate the Organ Systems
15.	Chapter 9: Structure and Integrative Functions of the Main Organ Systems
16.	Chapter 9: Structure and Integrative Functions of the Main Organ Systems
17.	Chapter 9: Structure and Integrative Functions of the Main Organ Systems
18.	Chapter 7: Processes of Cell Division, Differentiation, and Specialization
19.	Chapter 3: Transmission of Heritable Information from Generation to Generation and the Processes That Increase Genetic Diversity
20.	Chapter 3: Transmission of Heritable Information from Generation to Generation and the Processes That Increase Genetic Diversity

(Continued)

Item Number	Content Area
21.	Chapter 3: Transmission of Heritable Information from Generation to Generation and the Processes That Increase Genetic Diversity
22.	Chapter 3: Transmission of Heritable Information from Generation to Generation and the Processes That Increase Genetic Diversity
23.	Chapter 3: Transmission of Heritable Information from Generation to Generation and the Processes That Increase Genetic Diversity
24.	Chapter 3: Transmission of Heritable Information from Generation to Generation and the Processes That Increase Genetic Diversity
25.	Chapter 7: Processes of Cell Division, Differentiation, and Specialization
26.	Chapter 9: Structure and Integrative Functions of the Main Organ Systems
27.	Chapter 9: Structure and Integrative Functions of the Main Organ Systems
28.	Chapter 6: Structure, Growth, Physiology, and Genetics of Prokaryotes and Viruses
29.	Chapter 6: Structure, Growth, Physiology, and Genetics of Prokaryotes and Viruses
30.	Chapter 8: Structure and Function of the Nervous and Endocrine Systems and Ways in Which These Systems Coordinate the Organ Systems
31.	Chapter 9: Structure and Integrative Functions of the Main Organ Systems
32.	Chapter 9: Structure and Integrative Functions of the Main Organ Systems
33.	Chapter 9: Structure and Integrative Functions of the Main Organ Systems
34.	Chapter 9: Structure and Integrative Functions of the Main Organ Systems
35.	Chapter 9: Structure and Integrative Functions of the Main Organ Systems
36.	Chapter 3: Transmission of Heritable Information from Generation to Generation and the Processes That Increase Genetic Diversity
37.	Chapter 8: Structure and Function of the Nervous and Endocrine Systems and Ways in Which These Systems Coordinate the Organ Systems
38.	Chapter 4: Principles of Bioenergetics and Fuel Molecule Metabolism
39.	Chapter 9: Structure and Integrative Functions of the Main Organ Systems
40.	Chapter 5: Assemblies of Molecules, Cells, and Groups of Cells Within Multicellular Organisms
41.	Chapter 9: Structure and Integrative Functions of the Main Organ Systems
42.	Chapter 8: Structure and Function of the Nervous and Endocrine Systems and Ways in Which These Systems Coordinate the Organ Systems
43.	Chapter 9: Structure and Integrative Functions of the Main Organ Systems
44.	Chapter 9: Structure and Integrative Functions of the Main Organ Systems
45.	Chapter 2: Transmission of Genetic Information from the Gene to the Protein
46.	Chapter 3: Transmission of Heritable Information from Generation to Generation and the Processes That Increase Genetic Diversity
47.	Chapter 6: Structure, Growth, Physiology, and Genetics of Prokaryotes and Viruses
48.	Chapter 2: Transmission of Genetic Information from the Gene to the Protein
49.	Chapter 6: Structure, Growth, Physiology, and Genetics of Prokaryotes and Viruses
50.	Chapter 4: Principles of Bioenergetics and Fuel Molecule Metabolism
51.	Chapter 9: Structure and Integrative Functions of the Main Organ Systems
52.	Chapter 6: Structure, Growth, Physiology, and Genetics of Prokaryotes and Viruses
53.	Chapter 6: Structure, Growth, Physiology, and Genetics of Prokaryotes and Viruses
54.	Chapter 4: Principles of Bioenergetics and Fuel Molecule Metabolism
55.	Chapter 3: Transmission of Heritable Information from Generation to Generation and the Processes That Increase Genetic Diversity

Item Number	Content Area
56.	Chapter 5: Assemblies of Molecules, Cells, and Groups of Cells Within Multicellular Organisms
57.	Chapter 2: Transmission of Genetic Information from the Gene to the Protein
58.	Chapter 5: Assemblies of Molecules, Cells, and Groups of Cells Within Multicellular Organisms
59.	Chapter 4: Principles of Bioenergetics and Fuel Molecule Metabolism
60.	Chapter 2: Transmission of Genetic Information from the Gene to the Protein
61.	Chapter 2: Transmission of Genetic Information from the Gene to the Protein
62.	Chapter 5: Processes of Cell Division, Differentiation, and Specialization
63.	Chapter 2: Transmission of Genetic Information from the Gene to the Protein
64.	Chapter 8: Structure and Function of the Nervous and Endocrine Systems and Ways in Which These Systems Coordinate the Organ Systems
65.	Chapter 4: Principles of Bioenergetics and Fuel Molecule Metabolism

Chemical and Physical Foundations of Biological Systems

	Chapter in *McGraw-Hill Education: MCAT Chemical and Physical Foundations of Biological Systems*
1.	Chapter 15: Unique Nature of Water and Its Solutions Chapter 18: Structure, Function, and Reactivity of Biologically-Relevant Molecules
2.	Chapter 15: Unique Nature of Water and Its Solutions Chapter 18: Structure, Function, and Reactivity of Biologically-Relevant Molecules
3.	Chapter 17: Separation and Purification Methods
4.	Chapter 18: Structure, Function, and Reactivity of Biologically-Relevant Molecules
5.	Chapter 18: Structure, Function, and Reactivity of Biologically-Relevant Molecules
6.	Chapter 10: Translational Motion, Forces, Work, Energy, and Equilibrium in Living Systems
7.	Chapter 11: Importance of Fluids for the Circulation of Blood, Gas Movement, and Gas Exchange
8.	Chapter 12: Electrochemistry and Electrical Circuits and Their Elements
9.	Chapter 16: Nature of Molecules and Intermolecular Interactions Chapter 19: Principles of Chemical Thermodynamics and Kinetics
10.	Chapter 14: Atoms, Nuclear Decay, Electronic Structure, and Atomic Chemical Behavior
11.	Chapter 16: Nature of Molecules and Intermolecular Interactions Chapter 19: Principles of Chemical Thermodynamics and Kinetics
12.	Chapter 16: Nature of Molecules and Intermolecular Interactions Chapter 19: Principles of Chemical Thermodynamics and Kinetics
13.	Chapter 14: Atoms, Nuclear Decay, Electronic Structure, and Atomic Chemical Behavior
14.	Chapter 16: Nature of Molecules and Intermolecular Interactions
15.	Chapter 13: How Light and Sound Interact with Matter
16.	Chapter 13: How Light and Sound Interact with Matter
17.	Chapter 13: How Light and Sound Interact with Matter
18.	Chapter 13: How Light and Sound Interact with Matter
19.	Chapter 13: How Light and Sound Interact with Matter
20.	Chapter 16: Nature of Molecules and Intermolecular Interactions
21.	Chapter 18: Structure, Function, and Reactivity of Biologically-Relevant Molecules

(Continued)

Item Number	Content Area
22.	Chapter 13: How Light and Sound Interact with Matter
23.	Chapter 16: Nature of Molecules and Intermolecular Interactions
24.	Chapter 15: Unique Nature of Water and Its Solutions Chapter 16: Nature of Molecules and Intermolecular Interactions
25.	Chapter 16: Nature of Molecules and Intermolecular Interactions
26.	Chapter 16: Nature of Molecules and Intermolecular Interactions
27.	Chapter 14: Atoms, Nuclear Decay, Electronic Structure, and Atomic Chemical Behavior
28.	Chapter 16: Nature of Molecules and Intermolecular Interactions
29.	Chapter 14: Atoms, Nuclear Decay, Electronic Structure, and Atomic Chemical Behavior
30.	Chapter 11: Importance of Fluids for the Circulation of Blood, Gas Movement, and Gas Exchange
31.	Chapter 18: Structure, Function, and Reactivity of Biologically-Relevant Molecules
32.	Chapter 18: Structure, Function, and Reactivity of Biologically-Relevant Molecules
33.	Chapter 18: Structure, Function, and Reactivity of Biologically-Relevant Molecules
34.	Chapter 18: Structure, Function, and Reactivity of Biologically-Relevant Molecules
35.	Chapter 18: Structure, Function, and Reactivity of Biologically-Relevant Molecules
36.	Chapter 10: Translational Motion, Forces, Work, Energy, and Equilibrium in Living Systems
37.	Chapter 10: Translational Motion, Forces, Work, Energy, and Equilibrium in Living Systems
38.	Chapter 10: Translational Motion, Forces, Work, Energy, and Equilibrium in Living Systems
39.	Chapter 10: Translational Motion, Forces, Work, Energy, and Equilibrium in Living Systems
40.	Chapter 10: Translational Motion, Forces, Work, Energy, and Equilibrium in Living Systems
41.	Chapter 10: Translational Motion, Forces, Work, Energy, and Equilibrium in Living Systems
42.	Chapter 10: Translational Motion, Forces, Work, Energy, and Equilibrium in Living Systems
43.	Chapter 18: Structure, Function, and Reactivity of Biologically-Relevant Molecules
44.	Chapter 18: Structure, Function, and Reactivity of Biologically-Relevant Molecules
45.	Chapter 18: Structure, Function, and Reactivity of Biologically-Relevant Molecules
46.	Chapter 18: Structure, Function, and Reactivity of Biologically-Relevant Molecules
47.	Chapter 18: Structure, Function, and Reactivity of Biologically-Relevant Molecules
48.	Chapter 18: Structure, Function, and Reactivity of Biologically-Relevant Molecules
49.	Chapter 18: Structure, Function, and Reactivity of Biologically-Relevant Molecules

Item Number	Content Area
50.	Chapter 18: Structure, Function, and Reactivity of Biologically-Relevant Molecules
51.	Chapter 18: Structure, Function, and Reactivity of Biologically-Relevant Molecules
52.	Chapter 18: Structure, Function, and Reactivity of Biologically-Relevant Molecules
53.	Chapter 15: Unique Nature of Water and Its Solutions Chapter 16: Nature of Molecules and Intermolecular Interactions
54.	Chapter 15: Unique Nature of Water and Its Solutions Chapter 16: Nature of Molecules and Intermolecular Interactions
55.	Chapter 15: Unique Nature of Water and Its Solutions Chapter 16: Nature of Molecules and Intermolecular Interactions
56.	Chapter 15: Unique Nature of Water and Its Solutions Chapter 16: Nature of Molecules and Intermolecular Interactions
57.	Chapter 15: Unique Nature of Water and Its Solutions Chapter 16: Nature of Molecules and Intermolecular Interactions
58.	Chapter 16: Nature of Molecules and Intermolecular Interactions
59.	Chapter 15: Unique Nature of Water and Its Solutions Chapter 18: Structure, Function, and Reactivity of Biologically-Relevant Molecules
60.	Chapter 15: Unique Nature of Water and Its Solutions Chapter 18: Structure, Function, and Reactivity of Biologically-Relevant Molecules Chapter 19: Principles of Chemical Thermodynamics and Kinetics
61.	Chapter 18: Structure, Function, and Reactivity of Biologically-Relevant Molecules Chapter 19: Principles of Chemical Thermodynamics and Kinetics
62.	Chapter 15: Unique Nature of Water and Its Solutions Chapter 18: Nature of Molecules and Intermolecular Interactions
63.	Chapter 14: Atoms, Nuclear Decay, Electronic Structure, and Atomic Chemical Behavior
64.	Chapter 18: Structure, Function, and Reactivity of Biologically-Relevant Molecules
65.	Chapter 11: Importance of Fluids for the Circulation of Blood, Gas Movement, and Gas Exchange

Psychological, Social, and Biological Foundations of Behavior

	Chapter in *McGraw-Hill Education: MCAT Behavioral and Social Sciences & Critical Analysis*
1.	Chapter 10: Social Structure and Development: Theories of Social Structure
2.	Chapter 1: Vision: Higher Order Visual Processing
3.	Chapter 5: How Groups Affect Individuals
4.	Chapter 10: Social Structure and Development: Theories of Social Structure
5.	Chapter 9: Aggression/Altruism
6.	Chapter 6: Associative Learning: Operant Conditioning
7.	Chapter 6: Associative Learning: Operant Conditioning
8.	Chapter 6: Associative Learning: Operant Conditioning
9.	Chapter 6: Associative Learning: Operant Conditioning
10.	Chapter 6: Associative Learning: Operant Conditioning
11.	Chapter 7: Identity Formation
12.	Chapter 7: Identity Formation

(*Continued*)

Item Number	Content Area
13.	Chapter 7: Identity Formation
14.	Chapter 7: Identity Formation
15.	Chapter 7: Identity Formation
16.	Chapter 1: Vision: Rods and Cones
17.	Chapter 1: Vision: Rods and Cones
18.	Chapter 1: Vision: Rods and Cones
19.	Chapter 1: Vision: Rods and Cones
20.	Chapter 1: Vision: Rods and Cones
21.	Chapter 5: How Groups Affect Individuals
22.	Chapter 5: How Groups Affect Individuals
23.	Chapter 5: How Groups Affect Individuals
24.	Chapter 5: How Groups Affect Individuals
25.	Chapter 5: How Groups Affect Individuals
26.	Chapter 9: Romantic Attraction
27.	Chapter 9: Romantic Attraction
28.	Chapter 9: Romantic Attraction
29.	Chapter 9: Romantic Attraction
30.	Chapter 9: Romantic Attraction
31.	Chapter 4: Psychological Disorders: Types of Psychological Disorders
32.	Chapter 4: Psychological Disorders: Types of Psychological Disorders
33.	Chapter 4: Psychological Disorders: Types of Psychological Disorders
34.	Chapter 4: Psychological Disorders: Types of Psychological Disorders
35.	Chapter 4: Psychological Disorders: Types of Psychological Disorders
36.	Chapter 9: Romantic Attraction
37.	Chapter 9: Romantic Attraction
38.	Chapter 9: Romantic Attraction
39.	Chapter 9: Romantic Attraction
40.	Chapter 9: Romantic Attraction
41.	Chapter 10: Social Institutions
42.	Chapter 10: Social Institutions
43.	Chapter 10: Social Institutions
44.	Chapter 10: Social Institutions
45.	Chapter 10: Social Institutions
46.	Chapter 11: Demographic Structure of Society: Age
47.	Chapter 11: Demographic Structure of Society: Age
48.	Chapter 11: Demographic Structure of Society: Age
49.	Chapter 11: Demographic Structure of Society: Age
50.	Chapter 11: Demographic Structure of Society: Age
51.	Chapter 12: Healthcare Disparities
52.	Chapter 12: Healthcare Disparities
53.	Chapter 12: Healthcare Disparities
54.	Chapter 12: Healthcare Disparities
55.	Chapter 12: Healthcare Disparities
56.	Chapter 3: Stress/Chapter 4: Nervous System
57.	Chapter 3: Stress/Chapter 4: Nervous System
58.	Chapter 3: Stress/Chapter 4: Nervous System
59.	Chapter 3: Stress/Chapter 4: Nervous System
60.	Chapter 3: Stress/Chapter 4: Nervous System
61.	Chapter 2: Memory: Forgetting
62.	Chapter 2: Memory: Forgetting
63.	Chapter 2: Memory: Forgetting
64.	Chapter 2: Memory: Forgetting
65.	Chapter 2: Memory: Forgetting

MCAT

Practice Test 2

Biological and Biochemical Foundations of Living Systems

65 Questions   **Time Limit: 95 Minutes**

Questions 1–6 are based on the following passage.

Passage I

Maintenance of proper pH throughout the body is critical to homeostasis and is carried out through the collective efforts of multiple systems in the body. Failure of the kidneys or respiratory system can have drastic consequences on the body's ability to regulate blood pH. In order to regulate pH in the blood, a buffering system is used, which is shown. This reaction is completely reversible and is driven in either direction depending on the concentration of the reactants. A change to one item in this reaction will in turn affect the concentration of all of the other items. These reactions are catalyzed by the enzyme carbonic anhydrase:

$$CO_2 + H_2O \rightleftharpoons H_2CO_3 \rightleftharpoons H^+ + HCO_3^-$$

carbon dioxide   water   carbonic acid   bicarbonate ion

Generally, there are not many problems with the body's ability to have plenty of HCO_3^- ions in reserve. However, if HCO_3^- ion levels should become too low, the kidneys can generate more. In the distal convoluted tubule and collecting ducts of the nephrons, carbonic anhydrase converts CO_2 into H_2CO_3, which dissociates into H^+ and HCO_3^-. Kidney failure or damage to the carbonic anhydrase enzyme can cause major problems in the ability to regulate blood pH.

When the kidneys fail, their functions must be mimicked or death will occur. Dialysis is used as a means to perform some of the normal functions of the kidneys, which includes the maintenance of acid base balance. During dialysis, the patient's blood is exposed to dialysis fluid. The dialysis fluid has been prepared such that it will perform a variety of functions that include balancing blood pH, removing wastes from the blood, and removing excess fluids. While dialysis treatment is not nearly as efficient as natural kidney function, it can be used for extended periods of time in many patients with satisfactory results.

1. Based on the buffering equation shown in the passage, if H^+ ion concentration increased, which of the following would occur?
   A. The concentration of carbonic acid would increase.
   B. The concentration of carbon dioxide would decrease.
   C. Bicarbonate ion concentration would increase.
   D. Carbonic anhydrase activity would be reduced.

2. Increased levels of H_2CO_3 in the plasma should cause
   A. a decrease in ventilation rate
   B. an increase in ventilation rate
   C. an increase in plasma pH
   D. a decrease in the osmotic concentration of urine

3. Suppose plasma levels of carbon dioxide were elevated. On a cellular level, where does this carbon dioxide come from?
   A. It is produced during protein synthesis.
   B. It is a by-product of nucleic acid metabolism.
   C. It is a by-product of glucose metabolism.
   D. It is produced as a direct conversion from oxygen gas in the cells.

4. Many dialysis patients do not produce any urine, so dialysis must be used to manage their fluid levels. In order to remove excess fluids from the blood during dialysis, the patient's blood must be
   A. isotonic as compared to the dialysis solution
   B. hypertonic as compared to the dialysis solution
   C. hypotonic as compared to the dialysis solution
   D. the same pH as the dialysis solution

5. A class of drugs known as carbonic anhydrase inhibitors is known to increase the excretion of Na^+, K^+, and HCO_3^- ions via urine while allowing for the retention of H^+ ions. This should cause
   A. an increase in urine volume due to osmotic effects
   B. a decrease in urine volume due to increased water reabsorption at the distal convoluted tubule
   C. a decrease in urine pH due to the excretion of HCO_3^- ions
   D. no changes to the normal properties of urine since Na^+, K^+, and HCO_3^- ions are normally secreted in the urine

143

SECTION 1:
Biological and
Biochemical
Foundations of
Living Systems

6. One of the goals of dialysis is to remove several small, toxic solutes from the blood. In order for the toxins to move from the blood into the dialysis solution, which of the following processes must occur?
   A. active transport
   B. diffusion
   C. osmosis
   D. facilitated diffusion

Questions 7–12 are based on the following passage.

Passage II

Tuberous sclerosis is a genetic disorder characterized by the growth of benign tumors in the brain and on other organs of the body, including the heart, lungs, skin, and kidneys. The prevalence of the condition is about 1 in every 6000 newborns. The symptoms of the disease are variable in their severity, which may take years to fully develop and are often misdiagnosed. One common symptom seen in many tuberous sclerosis patients is kidney problems such as cysts. While the cysts typically cause no major problems, occasionally the cysts may bleed, which causes blood loss and anemia and may lead to kidney failure.

The disease is caused by mutations in two genes, tuberous sclerosis complex 1 and 2 (TSC1 and TSC2), although only one gene needs to be affected to have the disease. The TSC1 gene produces a protein called hamartin, while the TSC2 gene produces the protein tuberin. Both hamartin and tuberin act as tumor suppressors in the body. A typical pedigree for tuberous sclerosis is shown with affected individuals being shaded:

While most cases of tuberous sclerosis are acquired according to the pattern shown in the pedigree, some individuals acquire tuberous sclerosis through a process called gonadal mosaicism. In these cases, the parents do not have apparent mutations in TSC1 or TSC2 in their somatic cells, but they have passed the mutation to their children.

The prognosis for individuals with tuberous sclerosis depends on the severity of their symptoms. Some common symptoms are learning disabilities, seizures, mental retardation, skin abnormalities, and kidney failure. Most individuals with tuberous sclerosis live to a normal life expectancy.

7. Based on the pedigree provided, what is the most likely pattern of inheritance for tuberous sclerosis?
   A. sex-linked recessive
   B. sex-linked dominant
   C. autosomal recessive
   D. autosomal dominant

8. If an individual overexpressed both TSC1 and TSC2, you would expect
   A. that the individual would be likely to develop a severe case of tuberous sclerosis
   B. that the individual should develop a mild case of tuberous sclerosis
   C. that the individual would produce excess hamartin and tuberin to protect against tumor formation
   D. that the individual would produce minimal amounts of hamartin and tuberin, which would allow for some protection against tumor formation

9. In order for gonadal mosaicism to be the cause of tuberous sclerosis, a mutation must have occurred in the TSC1 or TSC2 gene during
   A. mitosis in embryonic development
   B. meiosis in embryonic development
   C. mitosis of brain and skin cells during childhood
   D. meiosis in at least one of the parents

10. Would two individuals who had tuberous sclerosis always have children with the disorder?
   A. Yes. If both parents have tuberous sclerosis, all of their gametes will contain mutated versions of TSC1 and TSC2.
   B. Yes. All children of parents with tuberous sclerosis should have the disease unless a spontaneous mutation occurs.
   C. No. It is possible that a child could inherit normal TSC1 and TSC 2 alleles from parents who have the disease.
   D. No. If both parents have tuberous sclerosis, their children will be carriers of the disease but will not display any symptoms of the disease.

11. An individual born with TSC as a result of gonadal mosaicism has parents that do not have the disease. If a pedigree of three or fewer generations were to be constructed for this individual and their family, the pattern of inheritance that would likely be suspected is
   A. sex-linked recessive
   B. sex-linked dominant
   C. autosomal recessive
   D. autosomal dominant

145

SECTION 1:
Biological and
Biochemical
Foundations of
Living Systems

12. Some tuberous sclerosis patients who develop kidney cysts are often undiagnosed until kidney damage or blood loss and anemia occur. Which of the following problems might a patient with anemia have?

   A. a reduced oxygen-carrying capacity

   B. a high hematocrit count

   C. an elevated erythrocyte count

   D. problems with blood clotting

Questions 13–18 are based on the following passage.

Passage III

The discovery and development of various types of anesthesia have revolutionized modern medicine, allowing many medical procedures to be performed with minimal discomfort to the patient. Local anesthesia is used to induce loss of sensation in a particular area, while general anesthesia is used to induce loss of sensation along with loss of consciousness. Both procaine (also known as novocaine) and lidocaine are drugs used for local anesthesia, and they have similar mechanisms of action. The drugs affect neurons in the local areas to which they are applied by preventing the opening of Na^+ gated channels in the neurons.

Procaine and lidocaine have their own advantages and disadvantages. For example, procaine has the ability to cause vasoconstriction in addition to its analgesic properties. However, lidocaine induces anesthesia faster and for a longer period of time than procaine. In addition to being used as an anesthetic, lidocaine is often used in the treatment of ventricular fibrillation, a condition where the cardiac muscle displays rapid, uncoordinated, and weak rhythms. The drug causes decreased excitability of the ventricles by blocking Na^+ gated channels, while the sinoatrial node in the right atrium is unaffected by the drug.

Procaine has a half-life of up to 0.5 hours in patients. When procaine is metabolized in the body, it is converted to para-aminobenzoic acid (PABA) in the plasma by the enzyme pseudocholinesterase, and PABA is then excreted by the kidneys. Lidocaine is twice as potent as procaine, but lidocaine is also twice as toxic. The half-life of lidocaine in patients is typically between 1.5 and 2 hours. Lidocaine is metabolized in the liver by two enzymes that produce the metabolites monoethylglycinexylidide and glycinexylidide.

13. If lidocaine is provided intravenously to a person with compromised liver function and a person with normal liver function, one hour later you would expect to see
   A. an increased plasma concentration of lidocaine in the patient with normal liver function as compared to the patient with compromised liver function
   B. a decreased plasma concentration of glycinexylidide in the patient with normal liver function as compared to the patient with compromised liver function
   C. an increased level of monoethylglycinexylidide in the urine of the patient with normal liver function as compared to the patient with compromised liver function
   D. all of the above

14. How would blocking gated Na^+ channels prevent the transmission of messages in nerves?
   A. If gated Na^+ channels are blocked, Na^+ concentrations remain higher inside the neuron than outside of the neuron.
   B. If gated Na^+ channels are blocked, the neuronal membrane cannot depolarize.
   C. Blocking Na^+ channels would prevent the Na^+/K^+ pumps from properly functioning.
   D. Blocking Na^+ channels would prevent neurotransmitters from binding to receptors at the synapse.

15. A neuron under the influence of an anesthetic such as lidocaine would MOST likely
   A. display decreased neurotransmitter release at the synapse
   B. show increased enzymatic degradation of neurotransmitters in the synapse
   C. show increased reuptake of neurotransmitters in the synapse
   D. display a more negative charge outside the neuron as compared to inside the neuron

16. Which type of neuron would be affected by lidocaine?
   A. motor neurons
   B. interneurons
   C. sensory neurons
   D. glial cells

17. What benefits would come from using an anesthetic such as novocaine, which causes vasoconstriction in addition to analgesic effects, during a surgical procedure?
   A. to keep blood pressure low
   B. to prevent infection
   C. to minimize bleeding during the procedure
   D. to prevent inflammation following the surgery

147

SECTION 1:
Biological and
Biochemical
Foundations of
Living Systems

18. The passage states that when lidocaine is given for ventricular fibrillation that the sinoatrial node is unaffected. The sinoatrial node normally functions as
    A. a valve in the heart
    B. the pacemaker of the heart
    C. the barricade between the right and left side of the heart that keeps oxygenated and deoxygenated blood from mixing
    D. a regulator of blood pressure in the heart

Questions 19–24 are based on the following passage.

Passage IV

Nitric oxide (NO) is a gas that plays important regulatory roles in mammalian processes as diverse as inflammation, blood flow, kidney function, and development. Nitric oxide is created from L-arginine using the enzyme nitric oxide synthase (NOS). In studies using mouse models, NO has been shown to be a critical regulator of early embryo development. Manipulation of NO in the mouse embryo at the two-cell stage of development can prevent further development of the embryo to the blastocyst stage of development.

In order to determine a more specific role for NO in early development, two-day mouse embryos (composed of two cells) were subjected to treatment by either sodium nitroprusside (SNP) or L-arganine methyl ester (L-NAME). Sodium nitroprusside is a NO donor, while L-NAME is a NOS inhibitor. In addition to a control group, three concentrations of SNP and three concentrations of L-NAME were tested. Each group consisted of 100 embryos. After the appropriate treatment, the number of embryos continuing to the blastocyst stage was counted and reported as follows:

Group	Treatment	Number of Embryos Reaching the Blastocyst Stage
1	Control	84
2	$0.1\,\mu$M SNP	88
3	$1.0\,\mu$M SNP	45
4	$10.0\,\mu$M SNP	0
5	$0.1\,\mu$M L-NAME	52
6	$1.0\,\mu$M L-NAME	35
7	$10.0\,\mu$M L-NAME	9

19. Which of the following would be the MOST appropriate treatment for the control group in this experiment?
    A. treatment with a known amount of SNP associated with a known value of NO needed to continue development
    B. treatment with SNP at a level lower than $0.1\,\mu$M
    C. treatment with L-NAME at a dosage higher than $10.0\,\mu$M
    D. treatment with neither SNP nor L-NAME

20. Based on the results of these experiments, which of the following conclusions is most strongly supported by the data?

   A. Minimal amounts of NO are optimal for development, but increased levels can be harmful.

   B. Increased amounts of NOS lead to the highest rates of embryo survival.

   C. The effects of L-NAME on development are not dose dependent.

   D. Increasing the inhibition of NOS is more detrimental to embryo development than increasing the amount of NO.

21. In order to further investigate the beneficial role of NO on early mouse embryo development, which experimental group should be further investigated?

   A. group 1

   B. group 2

   C. group 4

   D. group 6

22. Considering the fact that mouse development shares many similarities with human development, from which structure would the two-day-old embryos in this experiment be harvested?

   A. the uterus

   B. the vagina

   C. the oviducts

   D. the ovaries

23. Which of the following BEST characterizes the blastocyst stage of development?

   A. a solid ball composed of many cells that undergo mitosis

   B. a diploid, fertilized egg

   C. a ball of cells containing a fluid-filled cavity

   D. a loosely formed ball of cells that performs meiosis

24. Diabetics typically have lower levels of nitric oxide (NO) than individuals without diabetes. Low levels of NO can be associated with vascular inflammation and vascular damage, leading to reduced blood flow to extremities. Which of the following may help a diabetic patient?

   A. administration of L-NAME

   B. administration of SNP

   C. administration of L-NAME and SNP

   D. administration of SNP and an L-NAME antagonist

Questions 25–30 are based on the following passage.

Passage V

For many years, researchers have been interested in developing edible vaccines that would provide protection against various bacterial and viral diseases. An edible vaccine

149

SECTION 1:
Biological and
Biochemical
Foundations of
Living Systems

is a genetically modified organism (GMO) that is created when genes from the bacteria or virus being vaccinated against are inserted into plant cells. As the plants grow, they produce proteins from the bacteria or virus that the researchers are attempting to vaccinate against. When a person eats the plant, the viral or bacteria proteins serve as antigens, which initiates a primary immune response.

Some of the plants that are of interest in edible vaccine development are bananas, potatoes, tomatoes, corn, rice, tobacco, and soy beans. While early research focused on growing crops that produced edible products such as bananas, the most resent research is focused on extracting material from the leaves and seeds of the plants, dehydrating it, and putting it into capsules that can be swallowed. This allows for a more predictable dosage of the vaccine and eliminates concerns that the crops containing the vaccine would be accidentally eaten by individuals who are not in need of the vaccine. The term *edible vaccine* has now been replaced with the term *plant-derived oral vaccine*.

The development of plant-derived oral vaccines solves many problems associated with injectable vaccines. Because plant-derived oral vaccines are grown in crops, there is no problem with storage or refrigeration that is required of most traditional vaccines. These plant-derived vaccines also require no special training to administer. Additionally, when a vaccine is taken orally, it provides mucosal immunity due to the production of IgA antibodies by the immune system—in addition to systemic immunity. Since 90% of diseases enter the body through a mucus membrane, a vaccine that coerces mucosal immunity is of great benefit in the prevention of many diseases.

25. Suppose that an individual has been given a plant-derived oral vaccine against a specific virus. How could you determine whether the vaccine was effective?
    A. Test for the presence of interleukins in the blood of the patient.
    B. Test for the presence of interferons in the blood of the patient.
    C. Test to determine whether the complement system in the blood had been activated.
    D. Test for the presence of antibodies to the viral antigen.

26. In order to engineer a plant-derived oral vaccine, genes from the microbe to be vaccinated against must be placed into the plant genome. Which of the following choices would be the most reasonable way to achieve this goal?
    A. Perform polymerase chain reaction (PCR) to amplify copies of the bacterial or viral genes and then insert the copies into the plant cells by transduction.
    B. Insert the bacterial or viral genes of interest into a plasmid, which can serve as a vector to transfer the gene to the plant cell.
    C. Clone the genes into a bacterial cell and allow it to conjugate with a plant cell.
    D. Use DNA hybridization to allow the genes of interest from the bacterial or viral genome to hybridize with the plant DNA.

27. The goal of any type of vaccination is to induce active immunity without people getting ill from the disease that they are being vaccinated against. In order to have long-term effectiveness, the vaccine must cause the development of which type of cells in the immune system?
    A. cytotoxic T cells
    B. helper T cells
    C. plasma cells
    D. memory cells

28. When a vaccine is given orally, it must pass through the digestive system before being absorbed into the bloodstream, whereas injected vaccines enter the bloodstream directly. What problems might vaccine developers be concerned about with a plant-derived oral vaccine that has to pass through the digestive tract?
    A. There would be concern that the vaccine would not work quickly enough if it had to travel through the digestive tract.
    B. There would be concern that stomach acidity might damage the bacterial or viral proteins that were expressed by the plant cells of the vaccine.
    C. There would be concern that the vaccine might elicit an inflammatory response in the digestive tract.
    D. all of the above

29. Plant-derived oral vaccines produce bacterial or viral proteins that serve as antigens in the body. Which of these events would occur first when a new antigen enters the body?
    A. production of antibodies from plasma cells
    B. presentation of the antigen by a macrophage
    C. secretion of interleukin-2 from helper T cells
    D. attack of the antigen by cytotoxic T cells

30. A traditional vaccine that is administered either intramuscularly or subcutaneously would be expected to cause the formation of which type of antibodies initially following administration?
    A. IgE
    B. IgG
    C. IgM
    D. IgA

Questions 31–36 are based on the following passage.

Passage VI

Interleukins are cytokines or cell-signaling molecules. They come in many varieties and play numerous roles in modulating all aspects of the immune response. Interleukins are produced by many types of cells, and their secretion occurs rapidly, and typically

151

SECTION 1:
Biological and
Biochemical
Foundations of
Living Systems

briefly, as needed. Interleukins travel to target cells where they bind to receptors on the target cell, ultimately causing a cascade of events in the target that alter the behavior of that cell. Different types of microbes stimulate the release of different types of interleukins. The type of interleukins secreted will ultimately influence how the system responds to the infection.

An immunologist suspects that a recently discovered interleukin called interleukin X might be important in protecting against hepatitis C viral (HCV) infection. In order to test this possibility, two strains of mice are used—a knockout strain and a wild type strain. The strain of knockout mice used in this study has a loss of function mutation in the interleukin X gene. During the experiments to determine whether this new interleukin X might protect against HCV, the mice are exposed to an analog of HCV. Three weeks later, liver biopsies are taken from each of the mice. From the biopsied liver tissues, nucleic acids are extracted and polymerase chain reaction is used to detect the presence of HCV.

In the following data table, you will see data from 10 sets of mice in this experiment. A plus sign (+) indicates that PCR testing detected the presence of HCV and a minus sign (−) indicates that PCR testing did not detect the presence of HCV.

Animal Number	1	2	3	4	5	6	7	8	9	10
Wild type	−	+	−	−	+	−	−	−	−	−
Knockout	+	+	−	+	+	−	+	−	+	+

31. From the data presented, what can you conclude about the potential for this new interleukin X to protect against HCV infection in mice?
    A. The new interleukin provides no protection against viral infection.
    B. The new interleukin provides complete protection against viral infection.
    C. The new interleukin may provide some level of protection against viral infection.
    D. The new interleukin enhances viral infection.

32. Based on the data shown here, which of the following would provide support for the potential of the new interleukin X to prevent viral infection?
    A. finding that wild type mice tested negative for HCV in the presence of reduced interleukin X levels
    B. finding that knockout mice tested negative for HCV in the presence of supplemental interleukin X
    C. finding that knockout mice tested negative for HCV in the absence of supplemental interleukin X
    D. finding that wild type mice tested negative for HCV in the presence of increased interleukin X levels

33. In this experiment, the polymerase chain reaction is used as a means to detect the presence of the hepatitis C virus. How does this technique work?
    - **A.** Targeted primers bind to a specific nucleic acid sequence and amplify that target sequence, if it is present.
    - **B.** It uses primers specific to certain amino acid sequences to determine the presence of specific proteins.
    - **C.** It detects the presence of specific mRNAs to quantify the expression of specific genes.
    - **D.** It detects metabolic activity unique to the target organism it is attempting to detect.

34. Interleukins are just one of many immune modulators. In a typical viral infection, what other immune modulator would you expect to see secreted as part of the innate immune defenses?
    - **A.** interferons
    - **B.** antibodies
    - **C.** growth factors
    - **D.** complement proteins

35. The hepatitis C virus is a single-stranded RNA virus. A potential inhibitor of viral replication would include a substance that is antagonistic to
    - **A.** DNA polymerase
    - **B.** RNA polymerase
    - **C.** reverse transcriptase
    - **D.** DNA gyrase

36. Suppose that this newly discovered interleukin X is proven to be effective against viral infection. In which of the following cases would we expect an individual to test negative for the hepatitis C virus?
    - **A.** an individual with decreased expression of interleukin X
    - **B.** an individual with decreased expression of the receptor for interleukin X
    - **C.** an individual with increased expression of the receptor for interleukin X
    - **D.** an individual with a mutation in the receptor for interleukin X

Questions 37–42 are based on the following passage.

Passage VII

The process of quorum sensing is observed in a variety of species. It involves a system of communication between organisms that is dependent on population density. Bacteria are notorious for using quorum sensing (QS) via the secretion of secreted signaling molecules, called autoinducers (AI), to coordinate their gene expression once a threshold density of population is reached. Not only can bacteria communicate via QS within their species, but they can also cross-talk through QS between different

153

SECTION 1:
Biological and
Biochemical
Foundations of
Living Systems

species. In order to participate in quorum sensing, bacteria require a way to produce an autoinducer and a way to respond to autoinducers via binding to specific receptors.

One example of how bacteria use quorum sensing to their advantage is to regulate the gene expression of virulence factors. During infection, if a small number of bacteria were to express their virulence factors, this would largely have no impact on the host. Instead, bacteria wait until a quorum is reached in terms of population size, indicating that the population is large enough to express virulence factors. These virulence factors relate to such abilities as escaping the immune response, invasion, and spreading within the host.

We know that we are facing a current healthcare crisis related to the loss of effectiveness of many traditional types of antibiotics based on bacterial resistance. This provides a major impetus for identifying novel ways to target bacterial pathogens that avoid the use of antibiotics. Several chemical compounds and molecules have been identified as facilitators of quorum sensing inhibition. Typically, these factors can serve as signal-targeting enzymes or small-molecule inhibitors of signal synthases and receptors.

37. Autoinducers often act in positive feedback loops. This would mean that the production of an autoinducer would lead to
    A. the production of more autoinducer
    B. the production of less autoinducer
    C. upregulation of autoinducer receptors
    D. downregulation of autoinducer receptors

38. What sort of advantage would quorum sensing provide to bacterial populations as compared to the organisms within the population acting independently of one another?
    A. Quorum sensing allows bacteria to express genes collectively when the impact of those gene products will be maximized on their host.
    B. Quorum sensing allows individual bacteria to express a higher level of virulence than they could when acting in the absence of quorum sensing.
    C. Quorum sensing reduces the metabolic expenses for the majority of the population while increasing metabolic expenses for just a few members of the population.
    D. Quorum sensing allows members of a population to outcompete other populations for resources within the host.

39. Decreased density of a bacterial population should lead to
    A. increased expression of autoinducers
    B. decreased expression of autoinducers
    C. increased expression of virulence
    D. increased enzymatic degradation of autoinducers

40. Quorum sensing is used frequently within populations of bacteria such as *Pseudomonas aeruginosa* that form biofilms within their host. Once a quorum is reached, expression of the genes required for biofilm formation occurs. From the bacterial perspective, what direct advantage does the formation of biofilms provide?

    A. It provides a strong attachment to surfaces of the host.

    B. It enhances virulence expression of the organisms involved in the biofilm.

    C. It provides increased resistance to antibiotics.

    D. It enhances the secretions of toxins.

41. N-Acyl homoserine lactones (N-AHLs) are one type of autoinducer produced by certain species of bacteria. Different types of bacteria can produce N-AHLs with unique molecular structures by making minor changes to the core structure of the molecule. Given the structure of the molecule, what would be the most likely way they could do this?

    A. by altering the R group side chains

    B. by altering fatty acid chains

    C. by glycosylating the core structure

    D. by methylating the core structure

42. Targets of traditional antibiotics include all of the following EXCEPT

    A. ribosomes

    B. metabolic processes

    C. the cell wall

    D. the nucleus

Questions 43–48 are based on the following passage.

Passage VIII

Apoptosis, also known as programmed cell death, is initiated by a unique series of complex events in the cell. These events eventually result in the death of the cell and subsequent phagocytosis by macrophages. Apoptosis is a critical part of development as well as an important defense against cells that are damaged or present a threat to the organism.

One event that characterizes the initiation of apoptosis in the cell is apoptotic volume decrease (AVD). During AVD, the internal volume of the cell decreases due to mass water loss. The decreased volume of water in the cell creates an environment that is hospitable to the activation of enzymes needed to cause cell death. In order for the AVD to occur, there must be major changes to the polarity of the plasma membrane. These changes involve preventing K^+ intake and allowing a major influx of Na^+ into the cell that results in continued depolarization of the membrane. After this depolarization occurs, there is a release of cytochrome c from the mitochondrial membrane and an efflux of K^+ and other ions such as Na^+ and Cl^-. The eventual

155

SECTION 1:
Biological and
Biochemical
Foundations of
Living Systems

efflux of ions creates an osmotic gradient across the membrane. Water then follows the ions as they leave the cell that results in the AVD. It has been hypothesized that the major movement of water occurs through specialized and highly conserved proteins called aquaporins, which allow for regulated and fast movement of water out of the cell.

43. Based on the information provided in the passage, a drug that inhibited the activity of aquaporins would directly cause
    A. a decrease in ion efflux from the cell
    B. an increase in the osmotic gradient across the membrane
    C. a decrease in the AVD
    D. increased water loss via osmosis

44. Which of the following pieces of evidence would best support the hypothesis that aquaporins are in fact a critical part of the AVD event?
    A. finding no change in the AVD of a cell that has been engineered to overexpress aquaporins
    B. finding a decrease in the AVD of a cell that underexpresses aquaporins
    C. finding an increased AVD in a cell that does not express aquaporins
    D. finding no change in the rate of apoptosis in cells that have a mutation in an aquaporin gene

45. One of the early events required to initiate the AVD is continued depolarization of the plasma membrane. In order to cause continued depolarization of the membrane, which of these structures must be inhibited?
    A. Na^+/K^+ pumps
    B. voltage gated Na^+ channels
    C. K^+ leak channels
    D. Cl^- channels

46. During the AVD cytochrome c is released from the mitochondrial membranes. What process might be affected by the loss of cytochrome c?
    A. glycolysis
    B. fermentation
    C. Krebs cycle
    D. electron transport systems

47. Cells that perform apoptosis are ultimately able to activate enzymes within the cell that damage and destroy cellular contents. Which of the following organelles is MOST likely to become involved with apoptosis?
    A. the endoplasmic reticulum
    B. the Golgi complex
    C. lysosomes
    D. mitochondria

48. The best explanation for why water leaves the cell to initiate the AVD as the result of ion efflux is that
    A. the efflux of ions creates an isotonic solution outside of the cell
    B. the efflux of ions creates a hypotonic solution outside of the cell
    C. the efflux of ions creates a hypertonic solution outside of the cell
    D. the efflux of ions creates a solution conducive for active transport of water out of the cell

Questions 49–54 are based on the following passage.

Passage IX

Genetically modified (GM) foods contain DNA from more than one source. The goal of creating GM foods is to modify the organisms to express new and useful traits. A few examples involve engineering crops to be resistant to bacterial or viral infections, to be resistant to herbicides, to ripen more slowly, to survive extreme temperature changes, to contain vaccines, or to create crops that are more nutritious.

One GM food that has received media attention over the years is golden rice. This GM product was first introduced in 2000 and was engineered to provide carotene that is a precursor to vitamin A. The carotene in the rice provides the golden color. Vitamin A deficiency is a major problem in underdeveloped parts of the world, killing more than one million people a year, most of whom are children. This vitamin is critical for the development and maintenance of epithelial tissues, for vision, and for growth.

Rice plants normally produce carotene in the inedible parts of the plant. To be able to access and use the carotene, it was necessary to engineer the rice to produce it in the edible grains. In order to achieve this goal, two genes from daffodil plants, *psy* and *lyc*, and a bacterial gene called *crt1* were added to the rice genome. These genes engineered a pathway that produces lycopene, which is eventually converted to carotene. Each of these genes was placed under the control of a grain-specific promoter so that the products were produced in the rice grains.

While golden rice was produced to provide carotene, which the human body can convert into the essential vitamin A, the rice provided much less carotene than was anticipated. Golden rice 2, a modified version released in 2005, contains a much larger amount of carotene and, as such, is a better source of the vitamin. Field tests were conducted in 2009, and human consumption trials were completed in 2012. However, neither version has been grown in large-scale quantities at this time.

49. Genetically modified organisms can be produced in a variety of ways. In the case of golden rice, genes from the daffodil plant and bacteria were added to the rice genome. Which of the following would be necessary to remove the genes from these other organisms so that they could be added to rice?
    A. reverse transcriptase
    B. a viral vector
    C. restriction enzymes
    D. polymerase chain reaction

157

SECTION 1:
Biological and
Biochemical
Foundations of
Living Systems

50. The engineering of golden rice to have several exogenous genes that can be induced under the control of a single promoter would most resemble
    A. an operon system
    B. hybridized DNA
    C. a vector
    D. Okazaki fragments

51. When preparing GM organisms, it can be easier to get a eukaryotic cell to express bacterial genes than it is to get a bacterial cell to express eukaryotic genes. What might be the most reasonable explanation for this?
    A. Bacteria are more simplistic organisms, and it is more difficult to get them to express complex eukaryotic genes.
    B. The ribosomes of bacteria are different from eukaryotic ribosomes, and they have difficulty translating eukaryotic mRNA.
    C. Eukaryotic genes contain introns that must be spliced out prior to translation in order to make a functional protein. Bacteria lack the ability to perform RNA splicing.
    D. Bacterial cells recognize eukaryotic DNA as foreign and use nucleases to destroy it before it can be expressed.

52. An example of an epithelial tissue that might be produced and maintained by vitamin A would be
    A. epidermal tissue
    B. skeletal muscle
    C. adipose tissue
    D. bone

53. Genetically modified organisms, typically plants, are being developed as a means of administering vaccines. If these transgenic plants are to be successful as vaccines, they will need to
    A. stimulate inflammation in the recipient
    B. express antigens to stimulate adaptive defenses in the recipient
    C. contain antibodies to the organism being vaccinated against
    D. contain memory cells against the organism being vaccinated against

54. A typical GM organism would have _____ genes as compared to its non-GM organism equivalent.
    A. the same number of
    B. one or a few less
    C. one or a few more
    D. a lot more

Questions 55–65 are not associated with a passage.

55. The major constituent of blood plasma is
    A. protein
    B. NaCl
    C. water
    D. cholesterol

56. The hormone responsible for maintaining control of water balance in the human body is
    A. antidiuretic hormone
    B. luteinizing hormone
    C. adrenocorticotropic hormone
    D. growth hormone

57. The one principal effect *not* attributed to the hormone insulin is
    A. glycogen formation and storage
    B. conversion of glycogen into glucose
    C. carbohydrate oxidation
    D. inhibition of gluconeogenesis

58. Venous blood coming from the head area in humans returns to the heart through which major vessel?
    A. superior vena cava
    B. aorta
    C. hepatic portal vein
    D. carotid artery

59. During pulmonary gas exchange, oxygen and carbon dioxide always move
    A. into the alveoli
    B. into the blood
    C. from high to low concentration
    D. out of the blood

60. Prokaryotic and eukaryotic cells generally have which of the following structures in common?
    A. a membrane-bound nucleus
    B. a cell wall made of cellulose
    C. ribosomes
    D. linear chromosomes made of DNA

159

SECTION 1:
Biological and
Biochemical
Foundations of
Living Systems

61. A person is on medication to increase the pH of the stomach. A side effect is that the increased pH causes the normal stomach enzymes to be unable to function. Which component of this person's diet may NOT be completely digested?
    A. proteins
    B. nucleic acids
    C. fats
    D. carbohydrates

62. An extracellular matrix is characteristic of
    A. nervous tissue
    B. muscle tissue
    C. connective tissue
    D. epithelial tissue

63. Which of these statements BEST explains why your body prefers to perform aerobic respiration as opposed to anaerobic respiration?
    A. Anaerobic respiration does not allow for NADH to be recycled to NAD^+.
    B. Aerobic respiration requires less of an ATP investment than anaerobic respiration.
    C. Aerobic respiration produces far more ATP than anaerobic respiration.
    D. Aerobic respiration is easier for cells to perform than anaerobic respiration.

64. In Mendel's experiments with the pea plant, the gene for height exists in two allelic forms designated T for tall stature and t for short stature. In the second generation of a cross between a homozygous tall parent (TT) and a homozygous short parent (tt), the phenotypic ratio of dominant to recessive pea plants is
    A. 1:1
    B. 2:1
    C. 3:1
    D. 4:1

65. When a nonsteroid (peptide) hormone binds to a receptor on the cell surface
    A. the hormone moves into the nucleus where it influences gene expression
    B. the hormone-receptor complex moves into the cytoplasm
    C. a second messenger forms within the cell
    D. the cell becomes inactive

STOP. This is the end of Section 1.

Chemical and Physical Foundations of Biological Systems

65 Questions   **Time Limit: 95 Minutes**

Questions 1 and 2 are not associated with a passage.

1. Frogs are vertebrates that rely on their leaping ability for mobility and survival. Assuming frogs demonstrate a parabolic trajectory as they leap, which of the following graphs best describes the horizontal and vertical components of the velocity, v, of the frog as a function of time, t?

Horizontal component of velocity	Vertical component of velocity

2. To restore cardiac function to a heart attack victim, a cardiac defibrillator is applied to the chest in an attempt to stimulate electrical activity of the heart and initiate the heartbeat. Consider a cardiac defibrillator with a capacitor charged to approximately 6000 V. Assuming the capacitor has a capacitance of 30 μF, the energy released by the capacitor upon discharge of the defibrillator is
   A. 320 J
   B. 540 J
   C. 750 J
   D. 820 J

Questions 3–7 are based on the following passage.

Passage I

Amino acids are amphiprotic molecules; they contain a carboxylic acid group and a basic amino group. The structure of an α-amino acid can be represented by the structure:

$$R-CH-COOH$$
$$|$$
$$NH_2$$

There are 20 common amino acids, each with a different R group. The simplest one has $R = H$ and is called glycine. Glycine has two acidic protons. The carboxylic acid proton is more acidic. It has a pK_a of 2.4. Below this pH, it is protonated. Above this pH, it is in the carboxylate form.

The amino group has a pK_a of 9.8. Below this pH, it is protonated; above this pH it is in the form NH_2.

Every amino acid has a form called the zwitterion, which contains both a positive charge and a negative charge, and net zero charge. The pH at which the zwitterion exists is called the isoelectronic pH, or pI. The pI for a diprotic amino acid is found by taking the average of the pK_a's.

Experiment

A 50.0-mL sample of 0.050 M glycine was acidified to pH 2. Then it was titrated with 0.10 M NaOH. The pH was monitored continuously during the titration using a pH meter. The base was added in 1.0-mL increments until pH 3.0; then it was added in 0.30-mL increments until pH 8.0, when the volume of base added was changed to 1.0-mL increments once more. The pH was recorded after each increment was added, and the titration curve was drawn.

163

SECTION 2:
Chemical and
Physical
Foundations of
Biological Systems

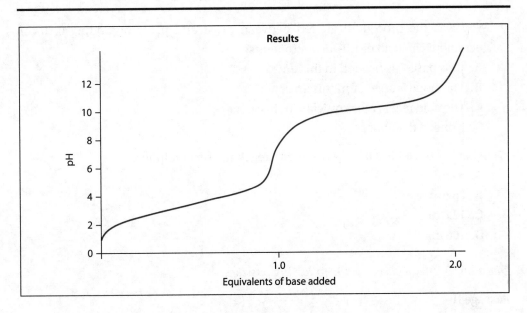

The flattish areas of the titration curve are called buffer zones. Here the pH does not change much upon addition of small amounts of acid or base.

Buffers are necessary in the body because all of our enzymes require a very narrow range of pH for maximum effectiveness.

3. There are two endpoints for this titration. The pH's for those points are
   A. 2 and 10
   B. 2 and 6
   C. 6 and 10
   D. 6 and 12

4. Which of the following BEST represents the structure of the molecule at pH 2?

   A. $R-CH-COOH$
      $\quad\quad|$
      $\quad\quad NH_2$

   B. $R-CH-COOH$
      $\quad\quad|$
      $\quad\quad NH_3^+$

   C. $R-CH-COO^-$
      $\quad\quad|$
      $\quad\quad NH_3^+$

   D. $R-CH-COO^-$
      $\quad\quad|$
      $\quad\quad NH_2$

5. At which of the given pH values does the zwitterion exist?
   A. pH 2
   B. pH 6
   C. pH 10
   D. pH 12

6. Why was the procedure altered between pH 3 and pH 8 by adding 0.30-mL increments instead of 1.0-mL increments?
   A. Less base was needed in this area.
   B. The slope is steeper in this area.
   C. The acid reacts more quickly in this area.
   D. None of the above

7. What volume of NaOH was needed to reach the first endpoint?
   A. 50 mL
   B. 25 mL
   C. 12.5 mL
   D. 100 mL

Questions 8–14 are based on the following passage.

Passage II

A motion sensor, a device that relies on sound to continuously determine the changing location of an object, is used to graphically display its motion in terms of velocity versus time and acceleration versus time graphs.

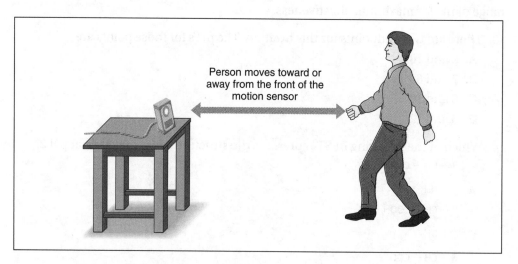

For example, if the person walks away from the motion sensor, the resulting distance versus time graph will be displayed:

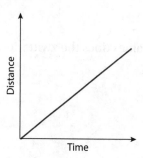

165

SECTION 2:
Chemical and
Physical
Foundations of
Biological Systems

The velocity of the person moving away from the motion sensor at the same rate can be determined by calculating the slope of the graph:

$$\text{velocity} = \text{slope of distance versus time graph} = \frac{\text{rise}}{\text{run}} = \frac{\text{change in distance}}{\text{change in time}}$$

The acceleration of the person can be determined in the same way by calculating the time rate of change of velocity.

A person performs the following series of movements in front of the motion sensor:

➤ Activity 1: Starting directly in front of the motion sensor, walk away from the sensor slowly, stand still, and then continue walking away from the sensor slowly.

➤ Activity 2: First standing still directly in front of the motion sensor, walk away from the sensor quickly, stand still, and then walk away from the sensor slowly.

➤ Activity 3: Standing approximately 3 meters in front of the motion sensor, walk toward the sensor quickly, stand still, and then walk away from the sensor quickly.

➤ Activity 4: Standing approximately 3 meters in front of the motion sensor, walk toward the sensor quickly; then move toward the sensor slowly and then stand still.

8. For the person standing directly in front and walking away from the sensor at a steady pace, the velocity versus time graph would be represented by which graph?

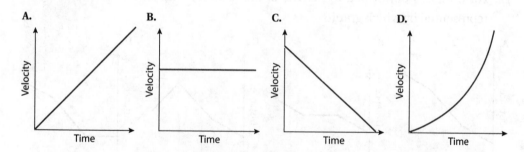

9. For the person standing directly in front of and walking away from the sensor at a steady pace, the acceleration versus time graph would be represented by which graph?

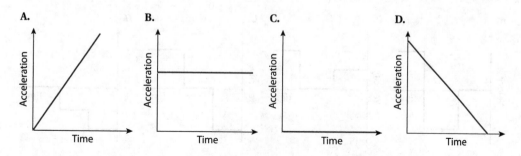

10. If the person were standing approximately 3 meters from the sensor and walked toward the sensor at a steady pace, the distance versus time graph would be represented by which graph?

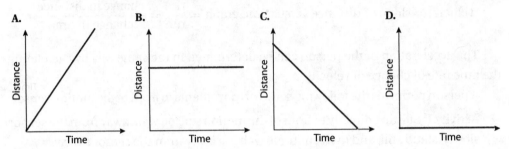

11. For the tasks performed in Activity 1, the distance versus time graph would be represented by which graph?

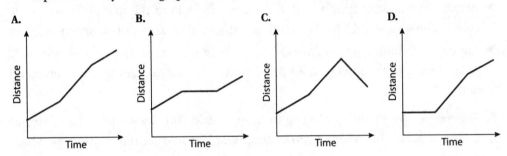

12. For the tasks performed in Activity 2, the distance versus time graph would be represented by which graph?

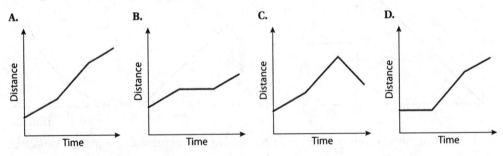

13. For the tasks performed in Activity 3, the velocity versus time graph would be represented by which graph?

167

SECTION 2:
Chemical and
Physical
Foundations of
Biological Systems

14. For the tasks performed in Activity 4, the velocity versus time graph would be represented by which graph?

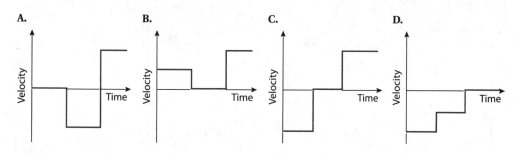

A.   B.   C.   D.

Questions 15–19 are based on the following passage.

Passage III

The following reaction was carried out according to the narrative experimental shown:

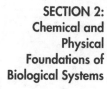

1   2

Substance	MW (g/mol)	d (g/mL)
Benzoic acid (**1**)	122	–
Thionyl chloride	119	1.631
(*S*)-2-methyl-1-butanol (**2**)	88.2	0.819
Dichloromethane	84.9	1.325
(*S*)-2-methylbutyl benzoate (**3**)	192	0.992

(*S*)-2-Methylbutyl benzoate (2). Benzoic acid (1.58 g) was dissolved in dichloromethane (20 mL) at room temperature. This solution was treated with thionyl chloride (1.04 mL) and allowed to stir for 45 min, after which (*S*)-2-methyl-1-butanol (1.19 mL) was added. After stirring for 1 h, the reaction mixture was transferred to a separatory funnel and washed with deionized water (30 mL). The organic phase was collected, dried over sodium sulfate, and concentrated in vacuo to give a crude mixture (1.92 g) that was analyzed by thin-layer chromatography (TLC 1), which showed the product was impure.

The crude mixture was dissolved in dichloromethane (30 mL), returned to the separatory funnel, and subjected to a second aqueous wash. The organic phase was collected, dried over sodium sulfate, and concentrated in vacuo to give a pure product (1.49 g) according to thin-layer chromatography (TLC 2). The pure product was also analyzed by IR spectroscopy.

15. When the crude reaction mixture was returned to the separatory funnel for a second aqueous wash, the aqueous phase MOST effective for providing a pure product would be
    A. deionized water alone
    B. 1 M hydrochloric acid
    C. 1 M sodium hydroxide
    D. saturated sodium chloride

169

SECTION 2:
Chemical and
Physical
Foundations of
Biological Systems

16. The yield of this reaction is
    A. 60% of theory
    B. 70% of theory
    C. 80% of theory
    D. 90% of theory

17. The IR spectrum most likely derived from the product of this reaction is
    A. Spectrum A
    B. Spectrum B
    C. Spectrum C
    D. Spectrum D

18. If the amount of (S)-2-methyl-1-butanol were increased, how would the rate of the reaction be affected?
    A. The rate would increase.
    B. The rate would decrease.
    C. The rate would be unaffected.
    D. It is impossible to predict the effect on rate.

19. The role of thionyl chloride in this reaction is to
    A. act as an acid catalyst
    B. act as a base catalyst
    C. convert the acid to a more reactive species
    D. convert the alcohol to a more reactive species

Questions 20–25 are based on the following passage.

Passage IV

A group of students were assigned the task of assembling a slingshot constructed from rubber bands secured with clamps at the edge of a tabletop that is a known distance, Δy, from the floor and then predicting the horizontal range distance, Δx, that a launched projectile (marble) will land from the base of the table. A schematic of the rubber band slingshot is shown in the following illustration:

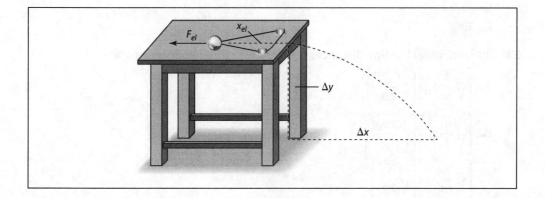

Before the slingshot was constructed, a series of measurements were performed on the rubber band to determine the stretching distance, x_{el}, as a function of an elastic force, F_{el}, applied to the rubber band. The data are shown here:

F_{el} (N)	2	3	4	5
x_{el} (cm)	14	21	26	30

The students used the data above to theoretically determine the landing distance of a marble. To compare the effectiveness of their theoretical calculations, the students then launched a marble by stretching the rubber band slingshot to four different values of x_{el}, and recorded the corresponding landing distances, Δx. The data are shown in the following table:

Stretch Distance, x_{el}	2.0 cm	4.0 cm	6.0 cm	8.0 cm
Predicted Value, Δx_{pr}	3.94 m	5.63 m	7.18 m	8.45 m
Observed Value, Δx_{ob}	2.64 m	4.55 m	6.01 m	8.04 m

20. The spring constant for the rubber band used as a slingshot is
    A. 18.8 N/m
    B. 1.88 N/m
    C. 0.188 N/m
    D. 0.0188 N/m

21. The velocity that the marble leaves the table upon release of the stretched rubber band is
    A. kmx_{el}
    B. $\dfrac{k}{m}x_{el}$
    C. $\sqrt{km}x_{el}$
    D. $\sqrt{\dfrac{k}{m}}x_{el}$

22. The percent error between the values collected for a stretch distance of 2.0 cm is
    A. 12%
    B. 26%
    C. 33%
    D. 42%

23. The horizontal landing distance, Δx, can be expressed according to
    A. $\left[\sqrt{\dfrac{k}{m}}x_{el}\right]\left[\sqrt{\dfrac{g}{2\Delta y}}\right]$
    B. $\left[\sqrt{\dfrac{m}{k}}x_{el}\right]\left[\sqrt{\dfrac{2\Delta y}{g}}\right]$
    C. $\left[\sqrt{\dfrac{k}{m}}x_{el}\right]\left[\sqrt{\dfrac{\Delta y}{2g}}\right]$
    D. $\left[\sqrt{\dfrac{k}{m}}x_{el}\right]\left[\sqrt{\dfrac{2\Delta y}{g}}\right]$

171

SECTION 2:
Chemical and
Physical
Foundations of
Biological Systems

24. If the students pull the slingshot back to 10 cm, the horizontal landing distance, Δx_{ob}, they might expect to see is
    A. 9.7 m
    B. 10.4 m
    C. 11.9 m
    D. 13.1 m

25. If the marble were doubled in mass, the effect on the horizontal landing distance would be
    A. decrease by $\sqrt{2}$
    B. increase by $\sqrt{2}$
    C. decrease by 2
    D. no change

Question 26 is not associated with a passage.

26. Which of the following is the MOST stable conformation of chlorocyclohexane?

    A.
    B.
    C.
    D.

Questions 27–31 are based on the following passage.

Passage V

Valine can be synthesized via the Strecker synthesis using isobutyraldehyde, as shown here:

In one particular synthesis, step 2 was incomplete, so a mixture of compounds 2 and 3 was encountered at the end. For purification, the reaction mixture was transferred to a separatory funnel and shaken with dichloromethane and 1M NaOH, after which the dichloromethane settled to the bottom.

27. In step 1 of the Strecker synthesis, isobutyraldehyde functions as a(n)
    A. oxidizing agent
    B. reducing agent
    C. nucleophile
    D. electrophile

28. Step 2 of the Strecker synthesis is best described as a(n)
    A. oxidation
    B. reduction
    C. hydrolysis
    D. condensation

29. The valine synthesized in the Strecker synthesis is best described as
    A. achiral and optically active
    B. achiral and optically inactive
    C. a racemic mixture and optically active
    D. a racemic mixture and optically inactive

30. In the separatory funnel, compound 2 is most likely
    A. charged and in the top layer
    B. charged and in the bottom layer
    C. neutral and in the top layer
    D. neutral and in the bottom layer

31. The best IUPAC name for compound 2 is
    A. 2-amino-3-methylbutanenitrile
    B. 2-cyano-3-methylpropanamine
    C. 2-(methylethyl)-2-aminoethanenitrile
    D. 1-cyano-1-(methylethyl)methanamine

Questions 32–34 are not associated with a passage.

32. In a direct current circuit, a voltage gradient, ΔV, generates and pushes current, I, through a wire of resistance, R, according to Ohm's law or $\Delta V = IR$. Ohm's law can analogously be applied to blood flow, Q, through a vessel of length, L, by the presence of a pressure gradient, ΔP. In this case, the variables involved in blood flow are related by Poiseuille's law or $Q = \dfrac{\pi r^4}{8 \eta L} \Delta P$. Given this, which of the following scenarios would result in the smallest resistance of blood flow?
    A. double the length and double the radius
    B. double the length and halve the radius
    C. halve the length and double the radius
    D. halve the length and halve the radius

33. For an individual who is myopic or nearsighted, the eyeball is longer than normal, causing visual images to be focused in front of the retina. Myopia can be corrected by
    A. using a concave lens, which increases the focal length
    B. using a convex lens, which increases the focal length
    C. using a concave lens, which reduces the focal length
    D. using a convex lens, which reduces the focal length

173

SECTION 2:
Chemical and
Physical
Foundations of
Biological Systems

34. Xenon-133, a radionuclide with a half-life of 5.25 d, is often used to assess pulmonary ventilation. If a dose of 28 mCi (millicuries) is administered to a patient in such a study, the radionuclide activity measured after 7 days is
    A. 1 mCi
    B. 5 mCi
    C. 8 mCi
    D. 11 mCi

Questions 35–39 are based on the following passage.

Passage VI

A student performed qualitative tests on a series of unknown chemicals in order to identify them. The unknowns included NaCl, NaHCO$_3$, sugar (C$_{12}$H$_{22}$O$_{11}$), MgSO$_4$, Na$_2$S$_2$O$_3$, cornstarch, and chalk (CaCO$_3$). These are all household chemicals. MgSO$_4$ is Epsom salts, NaHCO$_3$ is baking soda, and Na$_2$S$_2$O$_3$ is photographic fixer. The student was asked to identify six unknowns: A, B, C, D, E, and F.

The qualitative tests were based on the following:

➤ Solubility in water: starch is insoluble, as well as one of the other compounds. The rest are soluble in water.

➤ Chalk produces a gas when treated with acid.

➤ Starch turns blue when treated with iodine.

➤ MgSO$_4$ produces a milky precipitate when treated with aqueous ammonia.

➤ NaHCO$_3$ turns pink when treated with phenolphthalein.

➤ Na$_2$S$_2$O$_3$ decolorizes iodine solution.

➤ NaCl conducts electricity in solution.

➤ Sugar does not conduct electricity in solution.

The student prepared a flowchart that would aid in doing the experiments in a systematic manner and allow efficient identification of the unknowns.

Experiment

The experiments were conducted in the following order. The solubility of each chemical in water was tested first. From those results, the insoluble unknowns were tested next. The unknowns that were soluble in water were tested as aqueous solutions, rather than on the solid samples. First these solutions were treated with ammonia. Those that did not react with ammonia were tested further, with phenolphthalein and then iodine. From these results, the unknowns that had not reacted with any reagent were then tested for conductivity.

Results

Unknown	Solub	Conductivity	Acid	Phenolphthalein	NH_3	I_2
A	Y	Y	N	N	N	N
B	N	Y	Y	N	N	N
C	Y	Y	N	N	Y	N
D	N	N	N	N	N	Y_{BLUE}
E	Y	Y	Y	Y	N	N
F	Y	Y	N	N	N	$Y_{COLORLESS}$

From these results the student was able to identify all six unknowns.

35. Which of the following unknowns, when 1 mole was placed in enough water to make 10.0 liters of solution, showed the least increase in entropy?
    A. $NaHCO_3$
    B. $Na_2S_2O_3$
    C. $CaCO_3$
    D. $MgSO_4$

36. Unknown C was determined to be
    A. $NaHCO_3$
    B. $Na_2S_2O_3$
    C. $CaCO_3$
    D. $MgSO_4$

37. Unknown A was determined to be
    A. $CaCO_3$
    B. NaCl
    C. $Na_2S_2O_3$
    D. starch

38. The pK_a of the phenolphthalein used in testing the salts is 9.3. In a separate experiment involving a titration, phenolphthalein is used. For which of the following titrations is phenolphthalein best suited?
    A. Strong base with a weak acid
    B. Weak base with a strong acid
    C. Weak base with a weak base
    D. All of the above

39. The milky precipitate formed when $MgSO_4$ reacts with aqueous ammonia solution is $Mg(OH)_2$. Enough magnesium sulfate is used to saturate a solution that, when tested with a pH indicator strip, has a resulting pH of 10. What is the approximate K_{sp} of magnesium hydroxide?
    A. 10^{-12}
    B. 10^{-8}
    C. 10^{-4}
    D. 10^{-3}

175

SECTION 2:
Chemical and
Physical
Foundations of
Biological Systems

Questions 40–44 are based on the following passage.

Passage VII

Plants are able to perform all of the necessary functions and processes to maintain life through photosynthesis—the biochemical conversion of sunlight to the important nutrient, sugar, and the uptake of water through its roots. The uptake of water from the roots, through the stem, and into the tissue of the plant occurs via capillary action—the motion of fluid through extremely small vessels or tubes. Capillary action involves the interaction of the following two types of forces: adhesive forces that allow the water's molecules to adhere or stick to the plant tissues and cohesive forces that provide an attraction between water molecules. Upward movement of the water through the capillary vessels occurs when the adhesive forces are greater than the cohesive forces. The height, h, that the water will ascend up the plant depends upon the surface tension, T, of the water according to the equation:

$$h = \frac{2T}{\rho g r}$$

where ρ is the density of water ($= 1000 \, \text{kg/m}^3$), g is the acceleration due to gravity ($= 9.8 \, \text{m/s}^2$), and r is the radius of the plant stem.

To explore capillary action, the following experiment was conducted to determine the effects of sugar in water transported up the stem of identical carnation flowers. Three beakers were each filled with 0.5 L of water. One beaker (beaker 1) was set aside with no sugar added to the water. Fifteen grams of sugar was added to the water in the second beaker (beaker 2), and 30 grams of sugar was added to the water in the third beaker (beaker 3). Also added to each beaker were 10 drops of red food dye. A carnation was placed in each beaker and observed at 2-hour intervals, marking the height of the dye in the carnation stem. The data are presented in the following table:

Time (hr)	Height of Dye (cm) Beaker 1: No Sugar	Height of Dye (cm) Beaker 2: 15 g Sugar	Height of Dye (cm) Beaker 3: 30 g Sugar
0	0	0	0
2	2.41	0.32	0.15
4	4.17	1.69	0.8
6	5.93	3.06	1.45
8	7.69	4.43	2.1

40. Given that the radius of a carnation stem is 2.5 mm, the surface tension of the water required to reach a height of 8 cm is
   A. 0.01 N/m
   B. 0.1 N/m
   C. 1.0 N/m
   D. 10 N/m

41. The experiment showed that the dye in beaker 1 with no sugar traveled higher up the stem than the dye in beakers 2 and 3, each with increasing amounts of sugar placed in the water. What would be the best explanation for the results seen by the experiment?
    A. Weight of the water
    B. Length of the stem
    C. Size of the beaker
    D. Type of plant stem

42. For the carnation placed in beaker 3, the hourly rate of ascension of the dye up the carnation stem is approximately
    A. 0.13
    B. 0.28
    C. 0.69
    D. 0.95

43. For the carnation in beaker 1, the height that the dye will reach after 10 hours would be
    A. 7.8 cm
    B. 8.4 cm
    C. 9.7 cm
    D. 10.5 cm

44. For the carnation in beaker 2, how long would it take for the dye to reach 10 cm?
    A. 15 hours
    B. 16 hours
    C. 17 hours
    D. 18 hours

Questions 45–49 are based on the following passage.

Passage VIII

The treatment of 2-chlorohexane with sodium methoxide or sodium *t*-butoxide at 100°C leads to a mixture of products, including an S_N2-derived ether and two regio-isomeric alkenes (products of E2 elimination), as shown in the following diagram:

R	% Ether	% Terminal	% Internal
Me	35	22	44
t-Bu	10	79	11

177

SECTION 2:
Chemical and
Physical
Foundations of
Biological Systems

In both cases, alkene products dominate. However, when t-butoxide is used, the S_N2 product drops from more than a third of the reaction mixture to 10%, and the terminal alkene becomes the major product (versus the internal alkene in the case of methoxide).

45. Which property of t-butoxide (versus methoxide) is the most significant factor in the lower yield of ether?
   A. Higher pKa
   B. Increased steric bulk
   C. Decreased solvation
   D. Higher molar heat capacity

46. For the reaction with methoxide,
   A. the terminal alkene is the kinetic product and the thermodynamic product
   B. the terminal alkene is the kinetic product; the internal alkene is the thermodynamic product
   C. the internal alkene is the kinetic product; the terminal alkene is the thermodynamic product
   D. the internal alkene is the kinetic product and the thermodynamic product

47. For the reaction with t-butoxide,
   A. the terminal alkene is the kinetic product and the thermodynamic product
   B. the terminal alkene is the kinetic product; the internal alkene is the thermodynamic product
   C. the internal alkene is the kinetic product; the terminal alkene is the thermodynamic product
   D. the internal alkene is the kinetic product and the thermodynamic product

48. What would be the most reasonable product distribution from the reaction of 2-chlorohexane with isopropoxide at 100°C?
   A. 40% ether; 40% terminal alkene; 20% internal alkene
   B. 40% ether; 20% terminal alkene; 40% internal alkene
   C. 20% ether; 30% terminal alkene; 50% internal alkene
   D. 20% ether; 50% terminal alkene; 30% internal alkene

49. What would be the most reasonable product distribution from the reaction of 1-chlorohexane with methoxide at 100°C?
   A. 50% ether; 0% terminal alkene; 50% internal alkene
   B. 50% ether; 50% terminal alkene; 0% internal alkene
   C. 25% ether; 25% terminal alkene; 50% internal alkene
   D. 25% ether; 50% terminal alkene; 25% internal alkene

Questions 50–54 are based on the following passage.

Passage IX

Visible light is electromagnetic waves that travel at a constant speed of $c = 3.0 \times 10^8 \frac{m}{s}$ and range in wavelength from 400 nm (violet) to 700 nm (red). As light travels from one medium to another, light changes direction or refracts, a phenomenon that is important in image formation. All transparent media, such as air, water, glass, and oil, are characterized by an index of refraction, a value that indicates the amount by which the speed of light through that medium slows down. The index of refraction is defined as:

$$n = \frac{c}{v} = \frac{\text{speed of light in vacuum}}{\text{speed of light in medium}}$$

As light passes from one medium (medium 1) to another medium (medium 2), the angle of refraction of light through medium 2 (as measured with respect to the normal or vertical axis) is related to the angle of incidence of light through medium 1 through Snell's law of refraction:

$$n_1 \sin \theta_1 = n_2 \sin \theta_2$$

This is depicted in the following figure:

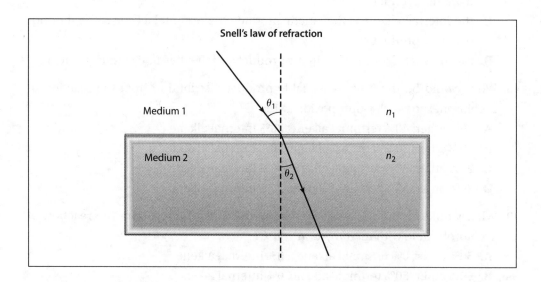

Refraction is important in image formation in the human eye. In the normal vision process, light passes through air ($n_{\text{air}} = 1.000$) and enters the eyeball through the cornea ($n_{\text{cornea}} = 1.376$), as shown in the following figure:

179

SECTION 2:
Chemical and
Physical
Foundations of
Biological Systems

Schematic diagram of the human eye

From the cornea, light enters the aqueous humor ($n_{\text{aqueous humor}} = 1.336$), passes through the lens of the eye ($n_{\text{lens}} = 1.406$), and enters a chamber filled with vitreous humor ($n_{\text{vitreous humor}} = 1.337$), where it then strikes the retina or the screen where the image is formed.

50. Red light of the visible spectrum has a wavelength of 700 nm. The frequency of red light is
    A. 2.0×10^{14} Hz
    B. 4.0×10^{14} Hz
    C. 2.0×10^{17} Hz
    D. 4.0×10^{17} Hz

51. The speed of light as it travels through the aqueous humor is
    A. $1.8 \times 10^8 \frac{\text{m}}{\text{s}}$
    B. $2.0 \times 10^8 \frac{\text{m}}{\text{s}}$
    C. $2.2 \times 10^8 \frac{\text{m}}{\text{s}}$
    D. $3.0 \times 10^8 \frac{\text{m}}{\text{s}}$

52. The speed of light is slowest when it passes through the
    A. aqueous humor
    B. lens
    C. cornea
    D. vitreous humor

53. If light is incident at 28° through air, the angle it is refracted through the cornea is
    A. 10°
    B. 14°
    C. 17°
    D. 20°

54. The majority of light refraction occurs in the human eye at the interface between
   A. air–cornea
   B. cornea–aqueous humor
   C. aqueous humor–lens
   D. lens–vitreous humor

Questions 55–60 are based on the following passage.

Passage X

The familiar 3% solution of hydrogen peroxide found in the local drugstore decomposes over time to form water and oxygen gas. The equation is:

$$H_2O_2 \text{ (aq)} \rightarrow 2H_2O \text{ (l)} + O_2 \text{ (g)}$$

As the oxygen forms, the mass of the liquid H_2O_2 decreases. The mass difference is equivalent to the mass of oxygen that forms. This reaction occurs very slowly but can be sped up by the addition of a catalyst such as I^-. One experimental method for determining the rate of the catalyzed decomposition of hydrogen peroxide requires measuring the mass difference over time intervals.

The molarity of the hydrogen peroxide solution at each interval can be calculated using a simple stoichiometry approach. The mass of oxygen is converted into moles, which is then multiplied by the ratio 2/1 to determine the moles of hydrogen peroxide that reacted. This value is then subtracted from the initial moles of hydrogen peroxide and then divided by the volume of the liquid sample.

To get the rate of reaction, a short time interval is used; the expression rate = $\Delta [H_2O_2]/\Delta t$ represents the instantaneous rate as t approaches zero.

Data		
Time (sec)	Mass O_2 Formed (g)	M H_2O_2
0	0	0.882
60	2.960	0.697
120	5.056	0.566
180	6.784	0.458
240	8.160	0.372
300	9.344	0.298
360	10.336	0.236
420	11.104	0.188
480	11.680	0.152
540	12.192	0.120
600	12.608	0.094

181

SECTION 2:
Chemical and
Physical
Foundations of
Biological Systems

When the molarity is plotted against the time, a logarithmic curve results that approaches M = 0 in an asymptotic fashion. At each point on the curve, the tangent represents the instantaneous rate of reaction. The rate constant for the reaction can be calculated using the rate equation

$\ln ([A]_0/[A]_t) = kt$

55. Which of the following statements is true?
    A. The instantaneous rate is fastest at the beginning of the reaction.
    B. The instantaneous rate is always faster than the average rate of reaction.
    C. The rate at the half-life is equal to one.
    D. All of the above

56. The rate over the first 60 seconds of reaction is
    A. 1.48 M/sec
    B. 0.349 M/sec
    C. 0.00308 M/sec
    D. 0.0116 M/sec

57. The rate constant for this reaction is
    A. [ln .882 – ln .697]/60
    B. [ln (.882 – .697)]/60
    C. [ln .697]/60
    D. [ln .882]/60

58. The half-life of this reaction is approximately
    A. 150 sec
    B. 190 sec
    C. 300 sec
    D. 450 sec

59. The decomposition of hydrogen peroxide follows first-order kinetics. This means that
    A. the rate is directly related to the hydrogen peroxide concentration
    B. the rate is directly related to the oxygen concentration produced
    C. the rate is logarithmically related to the hydrogen peroxide concentration
    D. the rate is logarithmically related to the rate constant

60. The catalyst I^- works to increase the rate of this reaction by
    A. changing the mechanism of the reaction
    B. lowering the enthalpy of the reaction
    C. raising the enthalpy of the reaction
    D. none of the above

Questions 61–65 are based on the following passage.

Passage XI

The two diastereomers of 1-bromo-2,2-dimethyl-4-(dimethylethyl)cyclohexane (compound 1) behave very differently when treated with lithium diisopropylamide (LDA). While both give 3,3-dimethyl-5-(dimethylethyl)cyclohexene (compound 2), the (1R, 4R)-isomer of compound 1 reacts much faster than the (1S, 4R)-isomer under the same conditions, as shown in the following diagram:

When compound 2 is treated with ozone, followed by dimethylsulfide, compound 3 is formed. Alternatively, when compound 2 is treated with borane, followed by basic hydrogen peroxide, compound 4 is formed, as shown:

61. The most reasonable mechanism for the first reaction (compound 1 > compound 2) is
    A. S_N1
    B. S_N2
    C. E1
    D. E2

62. The reason the (1R, 4R)-isomer reacts faster than the (1S, 4R)-isomer is
    A. in the (1R, 4R)-isomer, steric hindrance from the *t*-butyl group destabilizes the bromine
    B. in the (1S, 4R)-isomer, steric hindrance from the *t*-butyl group repels LDA
    C. the major conformer in the (1R, 4R)-isomer aligns dipoles so that it is more polar
    D. the major conformer in the (1S, 4R)-isomer lacks the proper orbital alignment

183

SECTION 2:
Chemical and
Physical
Foundations of
Biological Systems

63. Compound 2 is MOST accurately described as a
    A. single enantiomer exhibiting optical activity
    B. single enantiomer exhibiting no optical activity
    C. racemic mixture exhibiting optical activity
    D. racemic mixture exhibiting no optical activity

64. The most accurate structure for compound 3 is

    A.   *t*-Bu

    B.   *t*-Bu

    C.   *t*-Bu

    D.   *t*-Bu

65. The most accurate structure for compound 4 is

    A.   *t*-Bu

    B.   *t*-Bu

    C.   *t*-Bu

    D.   *t*-Bu

STOP. This is the end of Section 2.

Psychological, Social, and Biological Foundations of Behavior

65 Questions   **Time Limit: 95 Minutes**

Questions 1–5 are not associated with any passage.

1. In Dutton and Aron's "swinging bridge" study, which of the following was found to be a critical component of perceived attraction?
   A. Genetic factors influenced whom the participants found attractive.
   B. Childhood proximity and background were strong indicators of attraction.
   C. Lower adrenaline levels in response to more stable bridges were associated with increased attraction.
   D. Higher adrenaline levels in response to more unstable bridges were associated with increased attraction.

2. Kim has been in an automobile accident. He is unable to produce speech but is able to read, understand language, and even sing. Kim most likely has damage to which area of the brain?
   A. Wernicke's area
   B. Broca's area
   C. substantial nigra
   D. fusiform gyrus

3. Janey's family encourages her to continue her education. She works extremely hard and earns her master's degree in education. She is excited about beginning her teaching career and finally earning a paycheck. Her father, who is a school superintendent, arranges for her to have a job in an elementary school in his district. This is an example of which sociological construct?

   A. social mobility

   B. social stratification

   C. nepotism

   D. meritocracy

4. Robert is a salesman who sells jewelry door to door. His favorite sales technique involves showing his most expensive piece of overpriced jewelry to his potential customers. When the customer rejects the first piece, he displays a second, less expensive piece. Which of the following terms describes Robert's sales technique?

   A. door in the face

   B. foot in the door

   C. reciprocity

   D. ingratiation

5. According to sociological research, which of the following is true about increased mobility and globalization in society?

   A. As mobility has increased, more subcultures have developed because people are exposed to a greater number of diverse cultural influences.

   B. Mobility has had no impact on how people relate to their birth culture.

   C. As mobility has increased, residents of a particular area are less likely to retain traditional norms and customs that historically characterized the area.

   D. As mobility has increased, local residents are likely to become more intent on retaining traditional norms and customs to protect from external influences.

Questions 6–10 are based on the following passage.

Passage I

Researchers studying vision use various methods to investigate human perceptual experience. In certain instances the perceptual experience mirrors physiology. Research on spectral sensitivity of the rod and cone visual receptors highlights this relationship.

The following figure depicts the normalized absorbance of various wavelengths of light by each photoreceptor type. There are three types of cones that each respond preferentially to specific wavelengths in the electromagnetic spectrum. Rods also preferentially respond to specific wavelengths, overlapping the cone receptors' response frequencies.

187

SECTION 3:
Psychological,
Social, and
Biological
Foundations
of Behavior

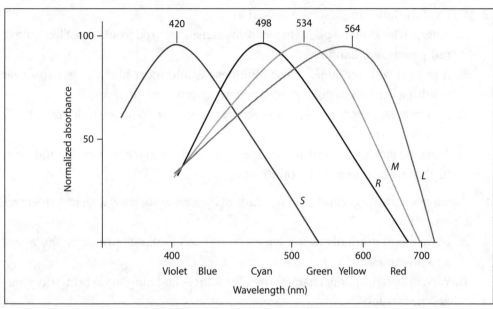

Four photoreceptor absorbance curves for each wavelength of light.

6. The three cone pigment curves shown in the figure are generally used to highlight which historical explanation for color vision?
   A. Hering theory of color vision
   B. opponent-process theory
   C. Young-Helmholtz theory of color vision
   D. Gestalt activation theory

7. A 600-mHz wavelength of light would excite which types of receptors?
   A. only S cones
   B. M and L cones
   C. M and L cones as well as R rods
   D. none of the above

8. Based on the graph and the trichromatic theory of color vision, which of the following statements is true?
   A. Light observed at 475 nm would most likely be perceived as cyan, and each type of receptor would be stimulated, with rods and red-sensitive (L) cones most stimulated.
   B. Light observed at 430 nm would most likely be perceived as blue, and each type of receptor would be stimulated, with rods and blue-sensitive (S) cones most stimulated.
   C. Light observed at 475 nm would most likely be perceived as cyan, and only cones would be stimulated, with blue-sensitive (S) and green-sensitive (M) cones most stimulated.
   D. Light observed at 430 nm would most likely be perceived as blue, and only cones would be stimulated, with blue-sensitive (S) and red-sensitive (L) cones most stimulated.

9. Which of the following statements is true?

    A. A person lacking rod pigment receptors sensitive to red would most likely have red-green color blindness.

    B. A person with red-green color blindness would most likely have a disorder resulting in a lack of color perception at the interneuron level.

    C. A person lacking cone pigment receptors sensitive to blue would most likely have red-green color blindness.

    D. A person lacking cone pigment receptors sensitive to red or green would most likely have red-green color blindness.

10. The wavelength of light and the amplitude of light are associated with what features in perception?

    A. Wavelength primarily characterizes color and amplitude primarily characterizes brightness.

    B. Wavelength primarily characterizes brightness and amplitude primarily characterizes color.

    C. Both wavelength and amplitude characterize color equally.

    D. Wavelength characterizes color, but amplitude has no impact on perception.

Questions 11–15 are based on the following passage.

Passage II

Evolutionary psychology has advanced our understanding of mate selection in humans. A prominent researcher, David Buss, conducted a number of research studies to investigate the evolutionary theory of mate selection in a wide range of cultures.

  The following data are a hypothetical adaptation of research looking at mate retention. The data are based on a study by Buss and Shackelford studying mate retention

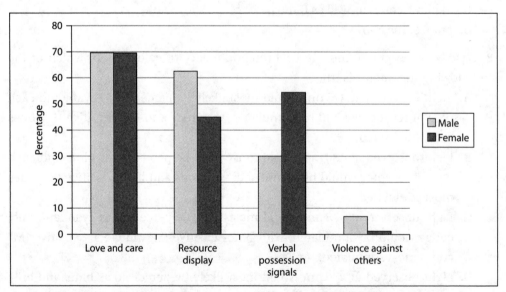

Mate retention tactics by sex. *Source*: Based on research conducted by D. M. Buss & T. K. Shackelford. "Vigilance to violence: Mate retention tactics in married couples." *Journal of Personality and Social Psychology*, 1997:72(2), 346.

189

SECTION 3:
Psychological,
Social, and
Biological
Foundations
of Behavior

strategies. Participants were asked about tactics that they have engaged in while in a relationship. Love and care are forms of comforting tactics. Resource display includes tactics such as buying presents. Verbal possession includes labels such as "wife" or "boyfriend" or other tactics announcing that a mate is spoken for in social situations. Violence against others represents physical aggression against other people perceived to be making advances toward one's mate. In the graph, the *y*-axis indicates the percent of participants indicating that have used the tactic. The *x*-axis represents the tactic, with the vertical bars indicating the different sexes.

11. Which of the following statements is true based on the data shown?
    A. Men are more likely to use all four tactics.
    B. Women are more likely than men to engage in violence against others.
    C. Men are more likely than women to use resource display.
    D. Women are more likely than men to use love and care.

12. Which of the following statements represents how evolutionary psychology interprets the results shown?
    A. Men are more likely to use resource display because women value financial status as a characteristic in a mate; high financial status means that a man can support offspring and increase their likelihood of survival.
    B. Men are more likely to use resource display because women like nice gifts from their mate.
    C. Men are more likely to use resource display because it proves that they are powerful, and women are more loyal to powerful men out of fear.
    D. Men are more likely to use resource display because it will attract multiple women; in that case, it is not a problem if a man loses his current mate.

13. Which of the following characterizes how males select mates, according to evolutionary psychology?
    A. Males select mates based mainly on financial status of their potential partner.
    B. Males select mates based mainly on the youth, attractiveness, and good health of their potential partner.
    C. Males select mates based mainly on the education and ambition of their potential partner.
    D. Males select mates based mainly on the industriousness of their potential partner.

14. Which of the following potential follow-up investigations would be most likely to contribute to further understanding of the mate selection process in humans, from an evolutionary psychology perspective?
    A. conducting the study on the same group of participants over time
    B. asking participants to complete a self-assessment and memory test
    C. asking participants to read relationship advice texts and testing them a year later to see if they show different responses
    D. investigating the correlation between behavior and the financial status and perceived attractiveness of the mates

15. If this study included a tactic called nonverbal possession signals (e.g., putting an arm around a spouse), according to evolutionary psychological theory, which gender would likely use this tactic more frequently and why?

   A. men, because nonverbal possession signals, like physical violence, are a form of physically protecting your mate from competitors

   B. men, because providing engagement and wedding rings to your spouse to wear as a nonverbal possession signal is another way to show competitors your level of resources

   C. women, because women often use public displays of affection to show how committed their mates are to them

   D. women, because nonverbal possession signals are another means to indicate possession without directly interacting with potential competitors

Questions 16–20 are based on the following passage.

Passage III

Researchers investigating implicit and explicit memory have found that certain disorders may impair explicit memory but not implicit memory. In a historic study, E. K. Warrington and L. Weiskrantz (1970) gave a list of words to amnesics and control participants. All participants then completed four memory tasks. Two were standard measures of explicit memory (recall and recognition tasks), and two were indirect measures of implicit memory in which the participants were asked to complete word fragments by guessing what the completed word or fragment was. Each memory task consisted of participants reading and later being tested on their implicit and explicit memory for a list of words.

The results of this study are shown in the following graph:

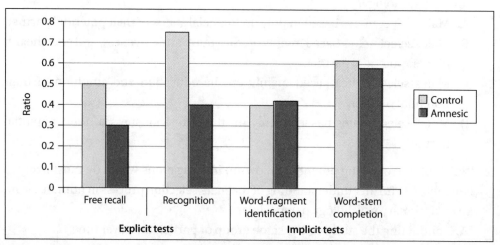

Amnesic and control participants completed four memory tasks. Two were explicit tests (free recall and recognition) and two were implicit tests (word-fragment identification and word stem-completion). *Source*: Adapted from E. K. Warrington & L. Weiskrantz. "Amnesic syndrome: Consolidation or retrieval?" *Nature*. 1970:228(5272), 628–630.

191

SECTION 3:
Psychological,
Social, and
Biological
Foundations
of Behavior

16. What does the graph most likely indicate about explicit versus implicit memory for amnesics compared to control participants?

    A. Amnesics perform worse on both explicit memory and implicit memory tasks compared to control participants.

    B. Amnesics perform equally well as control participants on explicit memory and implicit memory tasks.

    C. Amnesics perform better than controls on implicit memory tasks because there is no interference from explicit memories.

    D. Amnesics experience significant impairment for explicit memory tasks but do not experience significant impairment for implicit memory tasks compared to control participants.

17. Prior to Warrington and Weiskrantz's research, psychologists believed that amnesics lacked the ability to encode or store information in long-term memory. However, based on their research, what is the most likely explanation for the amnesics' difficulty performing specific memory tasks?

    A. Some amnesic participants are unable to remember new material but can access previously learned information to make judgments about current events.

    B. Some amnesic participants are able to learn new information (encoding) but are unable to explicitly state what they have learned (retrieval).

    C. Amnesic participants do not have any memory impairments when compared to control participants.

    D. Some amnesic participants are unable to learn new information but are able to explicitly recall lists of words.

18. If these results were examined using Endel Tulving's model of memory (episodic, semantic, procedural), which of the following statements is MOST likely to be true?

    A. Amnesic participants are able to encode and access semantic memory but are still impaired in their ability to retrieve the encoded information.

    B. Amnesic participants are able to encode and access episodic memory but are unable to access semantic memory.

    C. Amnesic participants have access only to procedural memories and therefore can only unconsciously follow scripts.

    D. Amnesic participants can encode and access episodic, semantic, and procedural memory with no impairments because these are part of a separate memory system.

19. Based on previous research, what is the brain structure that is most likely impaired in the amnesic population?

    A. cerebellum

    B. amygdala

    C. hippocampus

    D. Broca's area

20. Based on previous research, what is the brain structure that is most likely associated with the storage of long-term memory?
   A. amygdala
   B. hippocampus
   C. cerebral cortex
   D. Broca's area

Questions 21–25 are based on the following passage.

Passage IV

Research investigating different types of memory has found important differences between how those memories are recognized. The results of a hypothetical study are shown in the following graphs. In this study, during a training phase participants were instructed to listen to two separate study lists of musical sections, some familiar and some novel. Later, during a testing phase, participants listened to a mix including all of the initial melodies as well as an equal number of distractors. They were then asked to tell whether they had heard a melody during the training phase and, if so, which of the two study lists the melody was from.

Percent of familiar and novel melodies that were correctly identified as being from a specific study list.

193

SECTION 3:
Psychological,
Social, and
Biological
Foundations
of Behavior

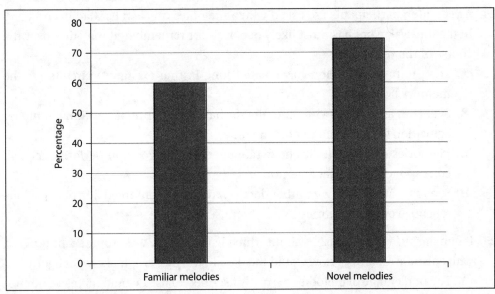

Percent of familiar and novel melodies that were correctly identified as being from one of the two study lists, but not a specific list.

21. Based on the results shown, which of the following is true about the data?
    A. Participants were better able to remember which list a melody was from than whether a melody had been heard during training.
    B. Participants were better able to remember which list novel melodies were from than familiar melodies.
    C. Participants were better able to remember which list familiar melodies were from than novel melodies.
    D. Participants were better able to identify familiar melodies than novel melodies as having been heard during training.

22. Based on memory research, which type of memory is most closely associated with list recognition performance?
    A. episodic memory
    B. semantic memory
    C. procedural memory
    D. implicit memory

23. Based on memory research, which type of memory is most closely associated with the data depicted for novel melodies in the second graph (percent correctly identified as being from one of the two study lists, but not a specific list)?
    A. episodic memory
    B. semantic memory
    C. procedural memory
    D. implicit memory

24. A year later, participants are asked which melodies on each list had been heard. In the interval, what has most likely occurred for remembered melodies over the course of the year?

    A. Long-term potentiation has created long-lasting excitatory circuits for the memory trace.

    B. Synapses associated with other details have been pruned, resulting in higher activation for the remembered melodies.

    C. Memories of the melodies have remained unchanged and performance will correspond to the intact memories.

    D. Synapses associated with other details have been reinforced due to conscious rehearsal of the memories.

25. If familiarity led to confusion about which list a melody was from (i.e., interfered with episodic memory), how would the data in the first graph likely change?

    A. The percentage of melodies correctly ascribed to list 1 would increase, but not the percentage correctly ascribed to list 2.

    B. The percentage of melodies correctly ascribed to list 2 would increase, but not the percentage correctly ascribed to list 1.

    C. The percentage of novel melodies correctly ascribed to both list 1 and list 2 would increase.

    D. The percentage of familiar melodies correctly ascribed to both list 1 and list 2 would decrease.

Questions 26–30 are based on the following passage.

Passage V

A classic study investigating observational learning was conducted by the psychologist Albert Bandura. In his study he explored whether children would model violent behavior after watching film sequences that featured violence.

In this study, four groups of child participants watched three different film sequences (aggressive-model-rewarded, aggressive-model-punished, and nonaggressive model control). In an additional control group, child participants were not shown a film.

➤ In the aggressive-model-rewarded group, the participants watched a film in which a child was rewarded for violent behavior toward another child.

➤ In the aggressive-model-punished group, the participants watched a film in which a child was punished for violent behavior toward another child.

➤ In the nonaggressive model control group, the participants watched a film in which there was no violent behavior between children.

195

SECTION 3:
Psychological,
Social, and
Biological
Foundations
of Behavior

The results of this study are shown in the following graph. Aggression is shown on the *y*-axis and the experimental and control groups are plotted on the *x*-axis:

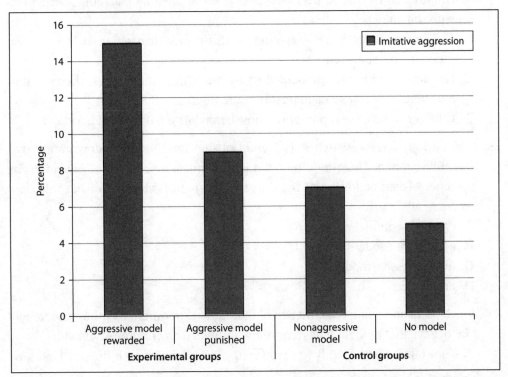

Modeling and aggression. *Source*: Adapted from a study by A. Bandura, D. Ross, & S. Ross. "Vicarious reinforcement and imitative learning," *Journal of Abnormal and Social Psychology.* 1961:67(12), 601–607.

26. Based on the graph, which of the following is true about imitative aggression?
    A. Children who view aggressive behavior and see the behavior rewarded are more likely to engage in imitative aggression.
    B. Children who view aggressive behavior punished are as likely as children who view aggression being rewarded to engage in imitative aggression.
    C. Children who view nonaggressive behavior are as likely as children who view aggressive behavior to engage in imitative aggression.
    D. Children are equally likely to engage in aggressive behavior regardless of whether they see behavioral models or no models at all.

27. According to Albert Bandura, this study highlights specific expectations concerning reinforcement and how reinforcement influences learning in children. In this view, which of the following is MOST probable based on the data from this study?
    A. Children learn how to perform specific novel tasks by engaging in the tasks with the models.
    B. Children passively learn how others perform specific novel tasks by watching others being punished.
    C. Children exhibit specific behaviors by modeling others when they see that another's behavior leads to positive outcomes.
    D. Children are able to report about how behaviors are displayed in others.

28. A second-grade class watches as a child pushes another child down and takes that child's lunch. The offending child is then put into a time-out (isolation) by a teacher. Which condition of Bandura's experiment is closest to what this class experienced?
    A. aggressive-model-rewarded
    B. aggressive-model-punished
    C. nonaggressive model
    D. no model

29. Which of the following is a criticism of Bandura's experiment by other researchers who believe that modeling has a minimal influence on children's behavior?
    A. The children in the study were too young to be definitively influenced by viewing films.
    B. In the study, the children in the control group displayed aggressive behavior similar to that displayed by the experimental groups.
    C. Child actors in the films were not aggressive enough in their depictions to produce violent behavior in child participants.
    D. The children in the study were in too artificial an environment and the tasks completed were not generalizable to real-world conditions.

30. Which of the following would MOST closely match the aggressive-model-rewarded condition of Bandura's study?
    A. Joey watches a friend play a violent video game in which punching small animals results in more points.
    B. Adam watches a feature film in which the lead character hits a pedestrian with his car and is sent to jail.
    C. Sally plays a video game that consists of solving problems using logic.
    D. Cameron watches a feature film showing parents grieving over the loss of a child.

Questions 31–35 are based on the following passage.

Passage VI

Education levels and frequent childbirth are linked to poverty levels. Worldwide organizations such as UNESCO and WHO track fertility rates, poverty levels, and education

197

SECTION 3:
Psychological,
Social, and
Biological
Foundations
of Behavior

across the world as countries experience both economic transitions (e.g., from agrarian to manufacturing) and increased globalization. On the following graphs, each dot represents a country's mean fertility rate plotted against the percentage of girls enrolled in secondary school and the percentage of the population living in poverty.

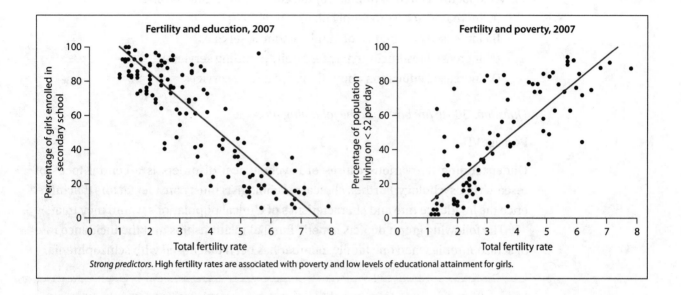

Strong predictors. High fertility rates are associated with poverty and low levels of educational attainment for girls.

31. Based on the graphs, in a country with an average fertility rate of six children per woman, what is the likelihood that a girl will be enrolled in secondary school, and what is the likelihood that she will live in poverty (<$2/day)?
    A. 41% chance of secondary enrollment; 83% likelihood of poverty
    B. 10% chance of secondary enrollment; 68% likelihood of poverty
    C. 5% chance of secondary enrollment; 68% likelihood of poverty
    D. 22% chance of secondary enrollment; 80% likelihood of poverty

32. Which of the following may explain why frequent childbirth alters women's social mobility?
    A. culture of poverty
    B. financial capital per family member
    C. social stratification
    D. increased human capital

33. Based on the graphs, if a man has four children, what is the likelihood that he will be living in poverty and what is the likelihood that he will have a secondary school education?
    A. 50% likelihood of poverty; 57% chance of secondary education
    B. 50% likelihood of poverty; education level unknown
    C. poverty level unknown; 57% likelihood of secondary education
    D. not enough information provided

34. What factor related to cultural capital could shift fertility levels?
    A. increased access to family planning services
    B. increased acceptance of family planning services
    C. increased resources to pay for family planning services
    D. increased education about family planning services

35. What factor related to human capital could shift fertility levels?
    A. increased access to family planning services
    B. increased acceptance of family planning services
    C. increased resources to pay for family planning services
    D. increased education about family planning services

Questions 36–40 are based on the following passage.

Passage VII

Understanding the various causes of psychological disorders is a central focus of research in psychology. Further, clinical psychologists must consider factors that influence the incidence rate and characteristics of clinical populations whom they treat.

The following graph depicts genetic familial relationships and the incidence rate of schizophrenia when one family member has been diagnosed with schizophrenia.

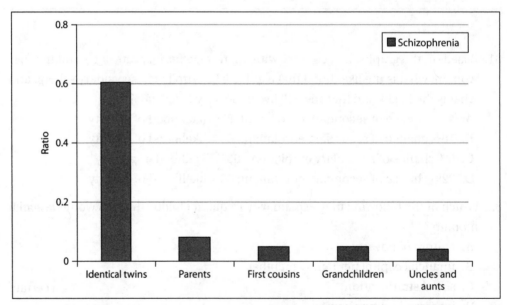

Familial relationship and incidence rate of schizophrenia when one family member is diagnosed with schizophrenia.

This second graph depicts the incidence rate of schizophrenia among children in relationship to each other and to parents when one or more family members have schizophrenia.

199

SECTION 3:
Psychological,
Social, and
Biological
Foundations
of Behavior

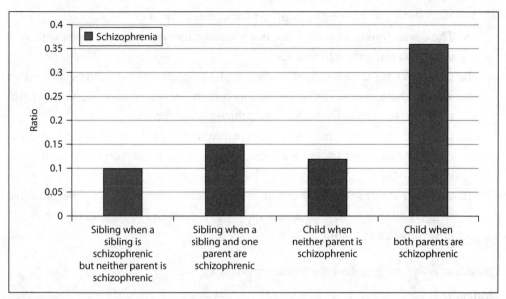

Parental schizophrenic status and incidence rate of schizophrenia diagnosis among other family members.

36. Based on the graphs, which group is at the highest risk for developing schizophrenia?
    A. children whose parents are both schizophrenic
    B. siblings with one schizophrenic parent
    C. individuals with uncles or aunts who are schizophrenic
    D. individuals with a schizophrenic identical twin

37. These data make the strongest argument for which view of the origin of schizophrenia?
    A. genetic causes
    B. environmental causes
    C. drug use/abuse causes
    D. both genetic and environmental causes

38. Which of the following is NOT associated with schizophrenia in the research literature?
    A. too much GABA or too much activity at the GABA receptors
    B. according to learning theory, family structure and social learning processes
    C. abnormally enlarged ventricles in the brain and reduced blood flow in certain portions of the frontal lobe
    D. sodium channels in specific neuronal pathways that are structured in an abnormal fashion

39. Based on the data in the graphs, which of the following would be the most appropriate follow-up study to investigate both heredity and environmental factors in schizophrenia?
    A. a survey of identical twins who grew up apart and those who grew up in the same household
    B. a survey of parents of schizophrenics about their childhood
    C. a survey of schizophrenics about the development of their disorder
    D. a survey of brothers and sisters who grew up in the same household

40. The data shown in the graphs imply which of the following?
    A. The development of schizophrenia is almost inevitable for children with parents or a twin with schizophrenia.
    B. Children who have family members with schizophrenia should be started on antipsychotic medications as soon as possible, even prior to showing symptoms, to reduce the likelihood of a schizophrenic break.
    C. Children who have family members with schizophrenia should avoid all stress because this could trigger a schizophrenic break according to the diathesis-stress model.
    D. Children who have family members with schizophrenia should be provided with additional environmental support to reduce the likelihood that they will develop schizophrenia.

Questions 41–45 are based on the following passage.

Passage VIII

Research into various states of consciousness has contributed greatly to our understanding about the mechanisms involved in human sleep. This research has provided insight into sleep as a restorative process and has highlighted the negative consequences of sleep deprivation.

The following figure depicts a full eight-hour sleep cycle. In the figure, sleep is divided into several stages based on EEG activity.

Sleep stages as a function of EEG activity during an eight-hour sleep period.

201

SECTION 3:
Psychological,
Social, and
Biological
Foundations
of Behavior

41. Based on the figure, which of the following statements is true?
    A. The amplitude of the EEG wave becomes smaller as deeper levels of sleep are reached.
    B. The length of REM sleep per sleep cycle generally increases as the night progresses.
    C. The length of time a person is in slow wave sleep increases as hours of sleep increase.
    D. The frequency of the EEG wave becomes greater as deeper levels of sleep are reached.

42. Most vivid dreaming occurs in which part of the sleep cycle?
    A. REM sleep
    B. stage 2 sleep
    C. slow wave sleep
    D. equally in all stages of the sleep cycle

43. Based on the figure, about how long is one sleep cycle?
    A. 20 minutes
    B. 4 hours
    C. 8 hours
    D. 90 minutes

44. Which two sleep states are associated with restorative processes?
    A. REM sleep and stage 2 sleep
    B. REM sleep and slow wave sleep
    C. stage 1 sleep and slow wave sleep
    D. stage 2 sleep and slow wave sleep

45. If Jose went to sleep at 10:00 p.m., at what time would he be most likely to be awakened by a car driving down the street?
    A. 2:00 a.m.
    B. midnight
    C. 1:30 a.m.
    D. 10:30 p.m.

Questions 46–50 are based on the following passage.

Passage IX

Research has examined how the presence of others affects how humans behave in different social contexts. This research has examined performance for different types of tasks and has also evaluated how group size affects performance. Studies have examined both internally motivated changes in behavior and losses due to coordination of activity with others (role duplication).

The following data represent a study conducted by B. Latane, K. Williams, and S. Harkins. In their study, they measured sound produced by individuals when asked to cheer or clap. They then manipulated the grouping conditions. Some individuals were alone, others were in actual groups of either two or six. Additional participants were told that they were placed into groups, but actually they were merely blindfolded and equipped with headphones (thus placing them in so-called pseudogroups). The decibels produced by each individual were measured for each condition. The results of this study are depicted in the following figure.

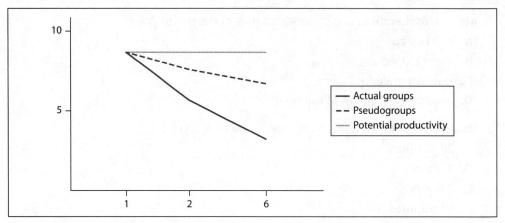

Loss of productivity based on group size and pseudogroup size. *Source*: Adapted from B. Latane, K. Williams, & S. Harkin. "Many hands make light the work: The causes and consequences of social loafing." *Journal of Personality and Social Psychology*, 1979:37(6), 822.

46. Based on the data shown, which of the following statements is true?
    A. Sound level increased the more participants there were in the groups.
    B. Sound level increased more in actual groups than in pseudogroups.
    C. Sound level decreased only when participants thought they were in a group but not when they were in an actual group.
    D. Sound level decreased for participants in actual groups and for participants in pseudogroups.

47. What would you expect to occur if the people in pseudogroups believed that the number of people in their groups was being altered?
    A. The decibel level would increase if the people in pseudogroups believed that there were more people in their groups.
    B. The decibel level would decrease if the people in pseudogroups believed that there were more people in their groups.
    C. The decibel level would decrease if the people in pseudogroups believed that there were fewer people in their groups.
    D. The decibel level would stay the same because there are not actually any more or any fewer people in the supposedly altered pseudogroups.

203

SECTION 3:
Psychological,
Social, and
Biological
Foundations
of Behavior

48. Based on research examining group productivity, what concept best explains the difference between the actual groups and the pseudogroups?
    A. loss of coordination
    B. the bystander effect
    C. social loafing
    D. group polarization

49. Based on research examining group productivity, what concept best explains the difference between potential productivity and the pseudogroups' productivity?
    A. loss of coordination
    B. the bystander effect
    C. social loafing
    D. group polarization

50. What are the implications for group projects based on these results?
    A. the larger the group size, the more social loafing will occur and the less effort each person will make toward completing a task
    B. the larger the group size, the more effort each person will make toward completing a task
    C. the smaller the group size, the greater the social diffusion of effort
    D. the larger the group size, the less effort any single person will need to contribute to reach a goal

Questions 51–55 are based on the following passage.

Passage X

Research investigating behavior in social situations has found that social behavior varies depending on the environment. Social behavior can involve either shallow acting or deep acting. Shallow acting requires altering facial expressions and body language so that on the surface, the individual conveys an emotion or opinion to conform to the social situation but does not really experience that emotion/opinion. Deep acting requires alteration of inner beliefs such that the individual believes the emotion or opinion he or she is expressing in order to conform to the situation.

In one study, deep acting and shallow acting in a social situation were examined for customer service workers. These workers routinely interacted with customers by smiling at them, speaking with them, responding to their queries, and detailing the benefits of various products. Later, stress was assessed for these workers.

Hypothetical results are depicted in the following figure.

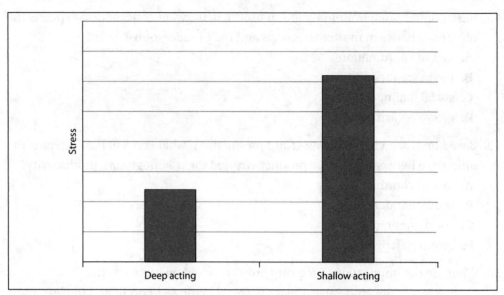

Perceived stress from social interactions involving deep acting and shallow acting.

51. Based on the results of this study, which of the following is true?
    A. Deep acting results in higher stress levels.
    B. Shallow acting results in higher stress levels.
    C. Stress levels are the same for both kinds of social behavior.
    D. Shallow acting is likely to be more common because it is easier.

52. Based on the dramaturgical approach of this study, and the data in the figure, which of the following is true of social interactions?
    A. The more social interactions that require shallow acting, the less perceived stress there will be.
    B. Social interactions should ideally not involve any acting.
    C. Social interactions involving deep acting should result in less stress.
    D. The fewer social interactions that require acting, the greater the stress will be.

53. According to cognitive dissonance theory, why would surface acting be more stressful than deep acting among customer service workers?
    A. Making sure that facial expressions and body language are consistent increases autonomic arousal and leads to elevated stress.
    B. Deep acting requires that you change your beliefs; therefore acting becomes less stressful.
    C. Individuals with social anxiety are more likely to engage in shallow acting.
    D. Deep acting provides more off-stage time compared to on-stage time.

54. Which of the following concepts involves an actor making sure that he or she chooses as an "audience" those people who will validate the actor's self-view?
    A. self-verification
    B. backstage self
    C. off-stage behavior
    D. self-referencing

205

SECTION 3:
Psychological,
Social, and
Biological
Foundations
of Behavior

55. According to the dramaturgical approach, when is an individual truly himself or herself?

    A. when the individual is alone (off-stage)

    B. when the individual has minimal interaction with others (on-stage)

    C. when the individual engages in self-talk dialogue (on-stage)

    D. when the individual engages in actions that cannot be seen by others (backstage)

Questions 56–60 are based on the following passage.

Passage XI

High levels of stress have been studied by a number of researchers. Research exploring stress and well-being has made some compelling discoveries. A common finding is that people who are under stress are more likely to report being sick than people who are under less stress. One such study by Hamrick, Cohen, and Rodriguez (2002) examined social connections and incidence of colds or flu. In their study, they asked participants about stressful events and about their social lives. Then they had the participants keep a diary for three months.

The accompanying figure shows the results of their study. The vertical bars on the *x*-axis represent participants who have either low or high levels of social contact, and who are under either low or high stress. The *y*-axis shows the percentage of participants who experienced a cold or flu.

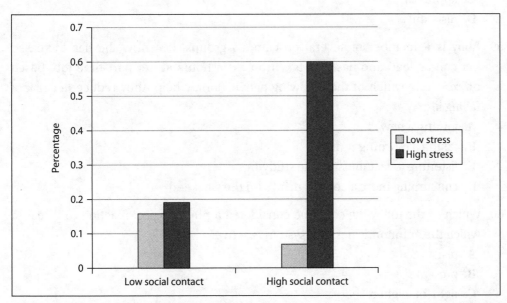

Participants were classified as either high-stress or low-stress and low-social-contact and high-social-contact groups. The percentage of the participants who experienced cold or flu is shown on the *y*-axis. *Source*: Adapted from N. Hamrick, Natalie, S. Cohen, & M. S. Rodriguez. "Being popular can be healthy or unhealthy: Stress, social network diversity, and incidence of upper respiratory infection." *Health Psychology*, 21.3, 2002:294.

56. What does this research indicate about high-social-contact vs. low-social-contact participants?
    A. High-social-contact participants under high stress are less likely to become sick than low-social-contact participants.
    B. High-social-contact participants under high stress are more likely to become sick than low-social-contact participants.
    C. Low-social-contact participants under high stress are less likely to become sick than high-social-contact participants.
    D. In general, high-social-contact participants are less likely to become sick than low-social-contact participants.

57. Based on the research depicted in the graph, which of the following is the MOST likely scenario that would contribute to the likelihood of a person becoming sick?
    A. giving a small birthday party for a family member
    B. getting a negative performance review on a minor job task
    C. dropping an expensive electronic device and having it break
    D. attending a large "new hire" orientation session for a major promotion in a new company

58. During a highly stressful time period, actions such as meditating or taking breaks to reduce or tolerate the stress are part of which strategy?
    A. accommodation
    B. coping
    C. appraisal
    D. resistance

59. Abby is a member of several on-campus groups. Recently, she has increased her course load and has also taken on extra hours at her part-time job. Based on research, which of the following activities may help Abby reduce her risk of falling ill?
    A. joining a new club
    B. taking a morning run
    C. listening to fast music while studying
    D. consuming more alcoholic drinks on the weekend

60. Which of the following could be considered a physiological reaction to threat in which the autonomic nervous system is active?
    A. resistance
    B. pressure
    C. fight-or-flight response
    D. appraisal

207

SECTION 3:
Psychological,
Social, and
Biological
Foundations
of Behavior

Questions 61–65 are based on the following passage.

Passage XII

Student performance has been assessed by sociologists as an indicator of how social structures function within a society. The following graph represents performance on standardized math tests by students in various US states, foreign countries, and one foreign city (Shanghai). The percentage of students considered proficient in math is shown on the *y*-axis.

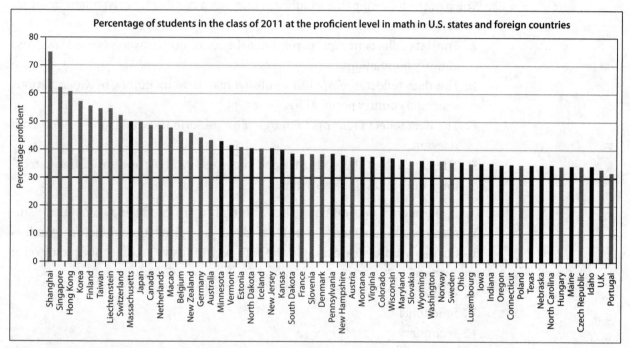

Percentage of proficient math students by country, city, or US state. *Source*: From P. E. Peterson, L. Woessmann, E. A. Hanushek, & C. X. Lastra-Anadón. "Globally challenged: Are US students ready to compete?" *Harvard's Program on Education Policy and Governance & Education Next, Taubman Center for State and Local Government, Harvard Kennedy School, PEPG Report,* 2011:11–103.

61. According to the data in the graph, which of the following is true?

   A. Students in the majority of listed US states score below students in the majority of listed countries in terms of math proficiency.

   B. Students in the majority of listed US states score above students in the majority of listed countries in terms of math proficiency.

   C. Students in the listed US states score the same as students in the listed countries in terms of math proficiency

   D. There is little difference in the math scores of students from the listed US states.

62. Based on the data in the graph, a sociologist is investigating how to maintain the differences in math proficiency between states and countries in order to preserve the distribution of manufacturing jobs in specific global regions. This approach is most closely related to which theoretical concept?
    A. conflict theory
    B. symbolic interactionism
    C. functionalism
    D. human theory

63. Which of the following BEST indicates one way a conflict theorist might interpret the data in the graph?
    A. The data reflect attempts to reinforce the status quo between various state and country populations.
    B. The data reflect attempts to reinforce historical inequities between various state and country populations.
    C. The data reflect attempts to marginalize performance indicators and are not relevant.
    D. The data reflect how countries and states use symbols and structures to reinforce individual characteristics.

64. Using these data, several countries with high math proficiency encourage students to become engineers in order to develop high-tech manufacturing industries. In this hypothetical example, the high-tech industries represent which level of production?
    A. primary
    B. functional
    C. secondary
    D. tertiary

65. Based on the graph, which of the following could be extrapolated about mathematics education?
    A. US culture does not value mathematical ability for girls as much as other cultures do.
    B. In recent years, the United States has fallen increasingly behind other developed countries in math and engineering education.
    C. Asian countries do not value mathematical training more than European countries do.
    D. Other US states would be well advised to copy successful aspects of mathematics education in the Massachusetts school system.

STOP. This is the end of Section 3.

Critical Analysis and Reasoning Skills

60 Questions   **Time Limit: 90 Minutes**

Directions: This section includes nine reading passages. Each passage is followed by a group of questions. Read each passage, and then select the one best answer to each question based on what you have read.

Questions 1–6 are based on the following passage.

Passage I

Sea beans. Ballast waifs. These adorable nicknames do not hint at the destructive nature of invasive plants. Sea beans are those plants whose seeds, buoyed by a pocket of air, float on the tide from one island to another, or even across vast stretches of ocean. Ballast waifs are less natural in origin; they are seeds that arrive on one shore from another in the soil placed in a ship's hold as ballast.

One remarkably lovely and dreadfully damaging ballast waif is *Lythrum salicaria*, the bright purple, spiky flower known commonly as purple loosestrife. Purple loose-strife is not a newcomer to US shores; it arrived from Eurasia, almost certainly via ship, some 200 years ago. It was widely used for medicinal and ornamental purposes throughout the nineteenth century. Its lovely purple blooms may still be seen in gardens throughout the country, where people love it for its long growing season.

For all its beauty, purple loosestrife is a menace. The same long growing season that makes it so beloved by gardeners makes it a seed-making machine. A mature plant may produce two or three million seeds a year.

That is not enough for *Lythrum salicaria*, however. It also propagates underground, sending out shoots and stems in all directions. It is also able to cross-pollinate with other species of *Lythrum*.

Scientists took little notice of purple loosestrife until sometime in the 1930s, when a particular strain began colonizing along the St. Lawrence River, an area rife with the sort of wetlands purple loosestrife likes best. Purple loosestrife does not just propagate wildly; it also adapts easily to changes in environment. As it starts up in a new area, it quickly outcompetes native grasses, sedges, and other flowering plants, forming dense stands of purple loosestrife where once heterogeneous wetland meadows existed. This not only eradicates the native plants, but it also removes food sources for migratory birds and other animals.

In recent years, purple loosestrife has had a devastating impact on native cattails and wild rice. It has invaded and destroyed spawning areas for fish. In rural areas, it is beginning to move away from wetlands and adapt to drier areas, encroaching on agricultural lands. In urban areas, it is blocking pipes and drainage canals. It has moved steadily westward and is now found in all states but Florida.

Attempts to control purple loosestrife have been only partially successful. It has proved resistant to many herbicides, and it is impervious to burning, as its rootstock lies beneath the surface and can reproduce from there. It can be mowed down and plowed under, and then replaced with a less invasive plant. This is very labor intensive in marshy areas that are substantially overgrown, but it may be the only way of eliminating the pest. Plowing it under requires unusually large discs on the plow because it is important to chop up the rootstock. Gardeners who have planted purple loosestrife are encouraged to dig it up and replace it with other, less damaging plants.

The best plan may be to seek a natural enemy of purple loosestrife, a weevil or insect that will destroy the plant. However, finding such an enemy that will target only purple loosestrife while leaving other, preferred plants intact is a daunting task. More important than that, introducing yet another foreign species to American swampland may lead to problems that make our purple loosestrife infestation look mild.

1. According to the passage, all of these are true EXCEPT
   A. purple loosestrife propagates through an underground system
   B. purple loosestrife has even affected the survival of fish
   C. purple loosestrife is best eradicated through controlled burning
   D. purple loosestrife is often used in American gardens

2. The mention of the St. Lawrence River shows primarily that
   A. sea beans prefer to travel on freshwater conveyances
   B. purple loosestrife does well in marshy areas along rivers
   C. most sea beans survive best in northern regions
   D. purple loosestrife can be replaced by less damaging plants

3. Which fact or facts about purple loosestrife add to its power of endurance?
   I. ability to cross-pollinate
   II. easy adaptability
   III. spiky stems and flowers
   A. I only
   B. II only
   C. I and II only
   D. I, II, and III

4. The author suggests that people enjoy growing purple loosestrife because it
   A. keeps out other weeds
   B. makes millions of seeds
   C. has a long growing season
   D. reduces weevils and insects

5. According to the passage, where would purple loosestrife easily thrive?
   I. in the subtropical swamps of central Florida
   II. in the wetland meadows of eastern Michigan
   III. along the inland waterways of North Carolina
   A. I only
   B. II only
   C. I and II only
   D. II and III only

6. According to the author, purple loosestrife can be eradicated by being mowed down, plowed under, and replaced with other species. Which of the following information, if true, would most WEAKEN this argument?
   A. *Lythrum salicaria* has been removed from some gardens through the careful use of an Australian slug.
   B. Replanted meadows where purple loosestrife once grew are slowly being taken over by a new, hardier strain of *Lythrum salicaria.*
   C. Cattails are coming back to some New York swampland once devastated by the incursion of *Lythrum salicaria.*
   D. Chopping up the rootstock of *Lythrum salicaria* with a plow adds an unexpected bonus in the form of nitrogen-rich fertilizer.

Questions 7–12 are based on the following passage.

Passage II

Since soldiers first formed armies, there has been martial music. It provided rhythm for drilling and marching, and it raised morale before battle and weakened that of the enemy during battle. From the war drums of Native Americans to the messenger drums of the early Chinese, from the trumpets of the ancient Egyptians to those of the ancient Celts, music has accompanied men into battle.

Fife and drum corps were popular from the Renaissance on, but the military band we think of today did not really exist until the eighteenth century, when brass instruments and woodwinds were combined in European bands to form a martial sound that could be heard even above the cannons and muskets of the battlefield. That sound was supplemented beginning in 1720 with the novel sound known as Janissary music.

The Janissaries were an elite corps of Turkish soldiers whose music was particularly suited to a military corps. Janissary music used kettledrums, cymbals, triangles, tambourines, and unusual forms of percussion such as the "Jingling Johnny," a tall, decorated pole hung with bells. By 1720, the sound had made its way to Europe by way of a gift from the Turkish sultan to the Polish army of Augustus II. Within a few years, Janissary percussion had been added to military bands in Russia, Austria, and Prussia. So-called "Turkish music" became wildly popular, and it did not take long for the lively military style to find its way into classical composition. This sudden craze presaged the Orientalism that would flavor European art in the next century.

Here in America, when we think of martial music, we think of John Philip Sousa and beloved marches on the order of "The Stars and Stripes Forever." However, 100 years earlier, Joseph Haydn used a Janissary style in his *Military Symphony No. 100 in G Major*, and Ludwig van Beethoven included a "Turkish March" in *The Ruins of Athens*. Wolfgang Amadeus Mozart based his opera *The Abduction from the Seraglio* on Janissary percussion. As the nineteenth century began, it became popular to add a "Janissary stop" to pianos and harpsichords, to provide a percussive accompaniment similar to that produced by the kettledrums of the Janissary corps.

As quickly as it had come, Janissary music passed out of favor, and by the middle of the nineteenth century, European and American bands had become formal, trained accessories to regiments, consisting typically of flute and piccolo, clarinets, oboe, saxophones, bassoons, horns, cornets, trombones, and percussion. In this country, the importance of martial music may have reached its peak during the Civil War, when every unit and regiment had its own small band. However, even today, according to *Mother Jones*, the Pentagon is the largest employer of musicians anywhere in the world, spending nearly $200 million of taxpayers' money annually on bands from Guam to Washington, DC—approximately 10 times what the federal government spends on K–12 music education. No longer do these bands follow men into battle, however; their purpose today is largely ceremonial, and you are more likely to hear them at a state funeral than at the rear of a forced march.

7. The author compares Native American drums to Chinese drums in terms of their
   A. tone
   B. appearance
   C. purpose
   D. value

8. In paragraph 4, the word *stop* is used to mean
   A. "period"
   B. "barricade"
   C. "interruption"
   D. "knob"

9. The discussion of Haydn and Mozart best illustrates the author's point that
   A. not all martial music is Janissary in flavor
   B. Janissary music was European in origin
   C. martial music influenced classical composers
   D. Orientalism affected painting as well as music

10. Which of the following assertions does the author support with an example?
    I. Janissary music used unusual forms of percussion.
    II. You might hear martial music at a state funeral.
    III. John Philip Sousa wrote beloved marches.
    A. I only
    B. II only
    C. I and III only
    D. II and III only

11. In the eighteenth century, enlisting in the army became known as "following the drum." If the author included this information in the passage, it would probably be used to
    A. support the notion that martial music was a critical part of military culture
    B. provide an example of idiomatic expressions based on music and art
    C. add details to the segment on the influence of martial music in the Civil War
    D. illustrate the change that followed the introduction of Janissary music

12. The author's mention of the level of funding provided for music education is most likely meant as a
    A. fascinating comparison
    B. critical comment
    C. humorous aside
    D. predictive claim

Questions 13–18 are based on the following passage.

Passage III

In the history of preemptive wars that end badly, we must consider the Zulu War of 1879. Like many wars of the nineteenth century, it was declared not by Parliament but rather by people on the scene. Sir Henry Bartle Frere was an emissary of the Queen, sent to Cape Town to find a way to unify the British and Boer colonies with a variety of independent black states to form a Confederation of South Africa. Standing in his way was the Zulu Army, a robust contingent of 40,000 warriors under the leadership of King Cetshwayo.

Frere looked for a way to seize Zululand. He used a series of minor border disputes to prompt an ultimatum to Cetshwayo, demanding that his army disband and be remodeled within 30 days. Cetshwayo refused to reply, which led to a state of war. A month and a half later, a British force invaded Zululand. They moved in three columns toward the royal compound.

On the 22nd of January, the middle column, led by Lord Chelmsford, a favorite of the Queen, split, with Chelmsford leading a large force to support a small reconnoitering party. The 1,750 left at camp soon found themselves surrounded by nearly 20,000 Zulus. Notice was sent to Chelmsford, but he would not be deflected from his plan. The resulting massacre at Isandhlwana reduced the middle column by 1,350 men. Some of the survivors retreated to Rorke's Drift, where they joined a small force of about 100 men who had successfully held off a few thousand warriors.

News of the massacre made its way to England, but Chelmsford, quite the modern military man, had already put a cover-up in place. He managed to convince the Queen and some of the press that Isandhlwana was overcome due to a lack of ammunition, and he put forth Rorke's Drift as a major victory, allowing that minor skirmish to be glorified as the massacre was all but forgotten. He would later blame Isandhlwana on the disobedience of an officer who died there.

Chelmsford's self-supporting propaganda was effective for a while, but as the Zulu War turned even bloodier, albeit more successful for the British, he was eventually recalled and replaced by Field Marshal Wolseley. Wolseley would command the British troops through the final campaigns of the Zulu War, campaigns that culminated in the capture of King Cetshwayo. The British divided up Cetshwayo's kingdom into 13 mini-chiefdoms, granting 11 to Zulus, 1 to a pro-British Basuto chief, and 1 to a white African mercenary. This plan led to many years of civil war, and in 1882, the British restored Cetshwayo to his throne, leaving his son in charge of a nearby territory. In 1883 that son joined with a band of Boer mercenaries and invaded his father's kraal, forcing his father into exile, where he soon died under mysterious circumstances. In league with the Boer who would become the first prime minister of South Africa, Louis Botha, a second son of Cetshwayo's attacked his brother and defeated his army. This son, Dinizulu, would be the last king of the Zulus to have any power. His land is now part of KwaZulu-Natal Province in South Africa.

13. In the context of the passage, the word *campaigns* means
    A. "races between candidates"
    B. "actions advancing a principle"
    C. "related military operations"
    D. "overland hunting expeditions"

14. The discussion of Rorke's Drift is used primarily to show
    A. why the capture of the king was a forgone conclusion
    B. how a minor success deflected attention from a major failure
    C. the many ways that British forces outmaneuvered the Zulus
    D. the use of British nomenclature to rename African landmarks

15. The passage suggests that the author would MOST likely believe that
    A. Chelmsford was a failure
    B. Chelmsford was a hero
    C. Frere was a hero
    D. Wolseley was a failure

16. Each of these at some time ruled some or all of Zululand EXCEPT
    A. a white African mercenary
    B. King Dinizulu
    C. Cetshwayo
    D. Lord Chelmsford

17. Which of these best shows that the British had little understanding of the land they occupied?

    I. Chelmsford initiated a cover-up of events at Isandhlwana.

    II. British forces moved in three columns toward the royal compound.

    III. The British plan for apportionment led to years of civil war.

    A. I only

    B. I and II only

    C. III only

    D. II and III only

18. The author's description of the Zulu War makes it seem most similar to

    A. the peasant uprising known as Kett's Rebellion

    B. the systematic genocide of the Nigeria-Biafra conflict

    C. the amphibious raid by the Allies on Dieppe, Normandy

    D. the removal by force of Saddam Hussein in Iraq

Questions 19 –25 are based on the following passage.

Passage IV

The man whom Franklin Delano Roosevelt christened "The Happy Warrior" in a nominating speech would later become a thorn in Roosevelt's side. Some thought the switch in loyalties was sour grapes, but others saw Alfred E. Smith as the epitome of William Wordsworth's "happy warrior" and therefore a man who "makes his moral being his prime care"—one who never made a move without consulting his conscience.

Alfred E. Smith was both a successful politician and an unsuccessful one. A four-term governor of New York State, he seemed a sure candidate for president, and indeed he ran three times for that position, only to lose each time.

He had several strikes against him. He was the Catholic son of Irish and Italian-German immigrants, making him anathema to nativists, the xenophobes who underwent a resurgence in the 1920s. He was from New York City, viewed even in the early twentieth century as disconnected from the national character. He was a progressive, which made conservatives of all stripes nervous. And he favored the repeal of Prohibition, a position that lost him the backing of many party leaders.

Who was this unlikely candidate? Born Alfred Emanuel Smith in 1873, Smith grew up on the Lower East Side of Manhattan. His father died when Smith was young, and the boy dropped out of school to take care of the family. At age 21, Smith supported a losing candidate in a local race and came to the attention of New York politicos, who took him under their wing. Nine years later, he ran successfully for the New York State Assembly, where he rapidly rose in the ranks to become majority leader and finally Speaker. He played a pivotal role in the revamping of New York's Constitution, was elected sheriff of New York County, and then ran for governor in 1918, winning handily. Although he lost a re-election bid two years later, he surged back in 1922 and would remain in the governor's seat for six more years. His terms were marked by unparalleled improvements in labor laws and laws protecting civil liberties, for Smith's goal was to support those he saw as most in need of government's assistance.

In this goal, he was allied with Franklin Roosevelt, and the two were close enough that Roosevelt nominated Smith for president in 1924. The Drys, or Prohibitionists, backed William McAdoo, a son-in-law of former President Woodrow Wilson. Smith's supporters and McAdoo's supporters were so far apart that finally a compromise candidate, John Davis, was nominated and promptly lost the general election to Calvin Coolidge.

In 1928, Smith received his party's nomination on the second ballot, but along with his anti-Prohibition leanings, his religion became a major issue during the campaign, paving the way for Herbert Hoover to win the general election. Meanwhile, Smith had arranged for the nomination of his New York colleague, Franklin Roosevelt, to be governor of New York. Although Smith lost his bid, Roosevelt did not.

Then came the Depression, and the election of 1932. Backroom dealings ensured that Franklin Roosevelt won the nominating process, with another would-be presidential candidate in the vice presidential spot on the ticket. Smith was left out in the cold on his third try for the presidency. Despite his former regard for Roosevelt, he began to work hard, if unsuccessfully, to defeat the New Deal. He supported two Republicans rather than Roosevelt in the 1936 and 1940 elections, and he died in 1944, a man who had never reached his desired goal, yet had inspired many of the changes for which his rival is now known.

19. One important argument of the final paragraph is that
    A. Roosevelt would have done better with Smith at his side
    B. the New Deal was anathema to someone with Smith's ideals
    C. Smith's background made him an improbable candidate
    D. Smith deserves credit for many of Roosevelt's successes

20. The passage implies that being from New York City is bad for a national candidate because
    A. urban candidates have trouble relating to those in the heartland
    B. New York is perceived as too different from the rest of the country
    C. westerners rarely support or give money to eastern candidates
    D. New York is the center of liberalism, but candidates must be neutral

21. The passage suggests that Roosevelt's change of heart toward Smith was influenced by
    A. ethics
    B. spitefulness
    C. miscommunication
    D. ambition

22. The mention of nativists shows primarily that
    A. only those born in the United States are eligible for the presidency
    B. bigotry figured into politics in the early twentieth century
    C. Prohibition was a critical issue for many urban voters
    D. a candidate for national office must embrace religion

23. According to the passage, why did John Davis win the Democratic nomination in 1924?
   A. He was not as far to the left as Smith.
   B. He was a Prohibitionist like McAdoo.
   C. He had the support of a former president.
   D. He was acceptable to Smith and McAdoo supporters.

24. The author's claim that Smith was a successful politician is supported by
   A. the explanation of his sobriquet, "The Happy Warrior"
   B. a review of his work in the Assembly and governor's office
   C. descriptions of his three runs for the presidency
   D. a list of the famous names that supported his candidacies

25. If Smith were to run for office today on a platform similar to his original plan, which of the following outcomes would MOST likely occur?
   A. He would be supported by Progressives and union leaders.
   B. He would be opposed by civil libertarians.
   C. He would be supported by those who favor immigration reform.
   D. He would be opposed by those who support social welfare programs.

Questions 26–32 are based on the following passage.

Passage V

The Shawnee people of the Ohio and Cumberland Valleys gave the American elk its other name, *wapiti*. Yet when we think of elk today, we rarely envision them as eastern animals. If we want to see elk in their natural habitat, we travel to Colorado or Montana, where they still roam the mountainous terrain.

Elk were, in fact, once found in the East, from Georgia north to New York and Connecticut. By the time of the Civil War, hunting and habitat destruction had caused their extinction in most eastern states. All of the eastern subspecies are now extinct. Elk County, Pennsylvania, and Elk County, Kansas, were without elk for more than a century.

At the beginning of the twentieth century, herds of elk in the Rocky Mountains faced death by starvation as encroaching farms depleted their winter feeding and finally the government decided to intercede. They gathered up elk from Yellowstone National Park and shipped 50 of them to Pennsylvania. The elk were to be protected, with no hunting of them allowed until eight years had passed.

At that early date, 1913, there was little understanding of the kind of acclimatization required when moving large animals from one habitat to another. The elk were released from cattle cars and chased into the wild to fend for themselves. Two years later, 95 more elk were moved from Yellowstone to Pennsylvania.

Elk are large animals with large ranges, and the damage these elk caused to corn-fields was substantial. The elk tended to move toward farming areas because that was where the food was. Farmers and poachers took some elk illegally, but the herds still began to grow. During the 1920s, several hunting seasons went by with harvests of one or two dozen elk, but then the numbers declined dramatically, and the elk were again put under protected status. No real census was taken until 50 years later, in 1971. At that time, according to the State Wildlife Management Agency, researchers found about 65 animals. Intensive work by the Bureau of Forestry to improve elk habitat, especially through reclamation of old strip mines, brought those numbers up to 135 by the early 1980s. By the year 2000, there were more than 500 elk in Pennsylvania, including many in Elk County.

In 1984 a group of hunters established the Rocky Mountain Elk Foundation, whose mission is to reintroduce elk in the states where they once roamed. The foundation runs into resistance from farmers and antihunting groups and generally requires majority approval from the community before animals are introduced. At present, new herds are established in Arkansas, Kentucky, Michigan, and Wisconsin in addition to Pennsylvania. There is talk of moving herds to Tennessee and to the Adirondack range in New York. It seems fairly clear that improving habitat for elk reintroduction improves conditions for other wildlife—wild turkey, whitetail deer, and black bear, among others.

Unlike the way things were done in the 1910s, today reintroduction is far more closely monitored and controlled. Animals are tested for disease. They are held in a large enclosure until they have acclimated to their surroundings. After a few weeks, they are released, but most have radio collars and/or ear tags that allow researchers to track their movements and habitat use. Research results help foresters know what to plant where in order to keep the herd healthy and help biologists know whether the herd is thriving or is in need of intercession. Land trusts are used to preserve habitat and to keep the elk from moving too close to cropland. The people in charge of elk reintroduction have no desire to live through another annihilation of the eastern *wapiti*.

26. According to this passage, a major early threat to elk populations was
    A. wolves and cougars
    B. vehicular traffic
    C. disease
    D. hunting

27. Based on information in the passage, about how many elk were moved from Yellowstone to Pennsylvania in the mid-1910s?
    A. 65
    B. 95
    C. 135
    D. 145

28. According to the passage, where might you see elk today?
    A. the Tennessee Valley
    B. Georgia
    C. the Adirondacks
    D. Arkansas

29. Which of the following assertions does the author support with an example or examples?
    I. New herds have been established in several states.
    II. Improving habitat for elk helps other wildlife.
    III. Land trusts are used to preserve elk habitat.
    A. I only
    B. III only
    C. I and II only
    D. I, II, and III

30. According to the passage, what is true of the elk in Pennsylvania today?
    A. They are the same as the elk who lived there 200 years ago.
    B. They are a different subspecies from the old Pennsylvania elk.
    C. They are a different subspecies from the elk found in the Rockies.
    D. They are only distantly related to the elk found in Yellowstone.

31. Which of the following findings best supports the author's contention that elk repopulation is carefully monitored?
    A. Farming to raise deer, elk, and reindeer is increasingly popular.
    B. Before 1997, there had not been a wild elk in Kentucky in 150 years.
    C. Rocky Mountain elk were among the original animals at the Hearst Zoo.
    D. Jackson County is testing potential elk herds for chronic wasting disease.

32. Which new information, if true, would most CHALLENGE the claim that elk reintroduction benefits other species as well?
    A. record sightings of wild turkey, pheasant, and grouse on reclaimed land in Pennsylvania
    B. surprising numbers of multiple births in moose from central and western Maine and New Hampshire
    C. a census showing that whitetail deer were migrating northward from Pennsylvania into New York
    D. an increase in temperature of one or two degrees in the headwaters of the Yellowstone River

Questions 33–40 are based on the following passage.

Passage VI

In linguistics, *metathesis* refers to the reversal of phonemes in a word. This can come about by accident, as in the common mispronunciation "aks" for *ask* or the common (and correct) pronunciation of *iron* as "i-orn." It may come about on purpose, as in various language games.

Accidental metathesis may be a process that takes place in the evolution of languages. Over time, for example, the Latin words *miraculum, periculum,* and *parabola* evolved into the Spanish words *milagro, peligro,* and *palabra*. Linguists posit that such changes usually occur when two consonants are of the same type, with similar mouth formations needed to create each one.

The Reverend Archibald Spooner, an Oxford dean, was known for his unintentional transpositions and gave his name to the particular metathesis he represented: *Spoonerisms*. Most famous Spoonerisms once attributed to Spooner are now believed to be apocryphal, but they are nevertheless amusing; for example, his supposed advice to a substandard student: "You have deliberately tasted two worms and will leave Oxford by the next town drain." Spoonerisms are funny when the metathesis involved changes one word into another, and they seem to lend themselves particularly well to off-color jokes.

Everyone is familiar with Pig Latin, in which initial consonant sounds are moved to the end of a word and followed with the syllable "ay." This is not pure metathesis, but it begins with the kind of metathesis known as backslang, in which syllables or letters in a word are reversed to produce a private code. Pig Latin may have begun as a language spoken in prisoner-of-war camps; it was certainly used in such camps during World War II and in Vietnam.

In Pig Latin, the phrase "Over the river and through the woods" becomes "Overay uhthay iverray anday oughthray uhthay oodsway." In other variations of Pig Latin, it might instead be "Overway unthay iverray andway oughthray uhthay oodsway." There are computer programs that translate from English to Pig Latin and back again, and there is even a version of the Bible written entirely in Pig Latin. For the most part, however, outside of prisoner-of-war camps, Pig Latin is a funny code used by children.

French children and teenagers use a similar code. Called *verlan* (a reversal of *l'envers,* or "reversal"), it is trickier than Pig Latin because it relies much more on phonetics than on spelling. In verlan, the word *café* becomes *féca,* but the word *tomber* ("to fall") becomes *béton*. Verlan becomes even more complex in words that end in silent *e* or which have only one syllable. While just a few words from Pig Latin have entered the vernacular (for example, *amscray* and *ixnay*), many verlan words are common lingo in France.

Historically, for reasons that are not quite clear, butchers have been frequent users of metathesis, creating their own backslang to converse without being understood by patrons. In France, this is called *louchébem* (*boucher,* or "butcher," with the first consonant moved to the end and the letter *l* placed in front). In Australia, it is known as *rechtub klat*. That name, of course, represents the ultimate in metathesis—the reversal of letters instead of merely syllables.

33. In the context of the passage, the word *transposition* refers to a
    A. reordering of letters or syllables
    B. movement of terms in an equation
    C. rendering into another language
    D. musical performance in a new key

34. Which of the following examples is presented as evidence that butchers are frequent users of metathesis?
    I. Spoonerisms
    II. *louchébem*
    III. Pig Latin
    A. I only
    B. I and II only
    C. II only
    D. II and III only

35. Which example(s) of metathesis does the author call accidental?
    I. verlan and other backslang
    II. *parabola* to *palabra*
    III. the pronunciation of *iron*
    A. I only
    B. II only
    C. I and III only
    D. II and III only

36. The discussion of prisoner-of-war camps shows primarily that
    A. Pig Latin can be entertaining even in difficult circumstances
    B. metathesis developed during the mid-twentieth century
    C. prisoners may revert to childish games to pass the time
    D. metathesis is useful and practical as a secret code

37. The author's claim that most Spoonerisms are apocryphal could BEST be supported by the inclusion of
    A. a list of transpositions attributed to the Reverend Spooner
    B. examples of modern-day transpositions based on famous Spoonerisms
    C. interviews with Spooner's contemporaries denying their authenticity
    D. Spooner's own letters to relatives, colleagues, and friends

38. Which of these might be an example of accidental metathesis?
    I. saying *interduce* instead of *introduce*
    II. saying *asterix* instead of *asterisk*
    III. saying *cause* instead of *because*
    A. I only
    B. I and II only
    C. II and III only
    D. I, II, and III

39. Based on information in the passage, which of these would be the verlan translation of *critique*?
    A. *euqitirc*
    B. *ticri*
    C. *tiquay*
    D. *quecriti*

40. The passage implies that Pig Latin is NOT pure metathesis because it
    A. does not transpose phonemes
    B. is not accidental
    C. includes the addition of an extra syllable
    D. does not add to the language

Questions 41–46 are based on the following passage.

Passage VII

Philosophers generally recognize three different conceptions of totality. Atomistic thinkers, such as Descartes and Wittgenstein, believe that the whole is no more than the sum of its parts. A thorough study of these parts, atomists believe, will lead to an understanding of the whole. A contrasting view, held by Schelling, Hegel (although some scholars question whether Hegel's ontology actually conforms to this formalist conception of totality), and members of the structuralist school of philosophy, holds that the whole has an identity of its own, separate from the nature of its component parts. A third view, and perhaps the most challenging to explore, is the dialectical/materialist idea of the whole held by Karl Marx. In this view, the whole is seen not simply as the sum of its parts as atomists believe or as something independent of its parts according to formalist thought. Instead, the whole is conceived of as the constantly changing and evolving interactions between all of its component parts.

In Marx's view, there are no things—static, independent objects or ideas—there are only processes. Everything that makes up the world is constantly in the process of becoming, with both its past and its future encapsulated in the very notion of the object itself. Furthermore, according to the dialectical materialist view, all objects are interdependent and the interactions they have with each other are also parts of their totalities.

Critics of this perspective point out, somewhat justifiably, that such an ontology has a number of difficulties. One of their major objections is that dialectical materialism is impractical to employ in any meaningful way. Consider how thinking of even a simple object such as a chair in this way quickly leads to a surfeit of information, connections, and processes. For a chair is not simply a chair, but the result of the labor of an individual, a process of manufacturing, the needs of a society that requires chairs, and many other factors. And each of these factors has its own past (and future) and myriad other connections as well. The number of relationships increases exponentially, which quickly makes a dialectical worldview utterly overwhelming to even the most agile philosophical mind.

Marxist philosophers attempt to work around this potential pathology by invoking what is called the process of abstraction. Abstraction allows the philosopher to draw certain boundaries around the object, idea, or relationship studied. Typically, these abstractions involve deciding an appropriate time scale to consider, the level of generality necessary for understanding specific interactions, and the vantage point from which to view a particular object of study. Abstraction on these levels allows the philosopher to bring certain relationships and processes into greater focus in order to understand them, while always keeping in mind that such an abstraction necessarily obscures various other connections. Marx famously used this process in his study of capitalism, sometimes viewing the system from the vantage point of the capitalist, other times assuming the perch of the worker and even at times trying to view the system from the perspective of capital itself. Similarly, sometimes Marx generalized people as simply members of their class in order to gain a better grasp of the relationship between owner and worker. Each new abstraction adds to the understanding of the system, and the process of abstraction must happen again and again in order to bring hidden connections into view.

41. The passage suggests that philosophical conceptions of totality
    A. have evolved over time from an atomistic view to a dialectical view
    B. have prevented philosophers from grasping the inherent connections involved in all things
    C. are based on three mutually exclusive conceptions of the relationships between part and whole
    D. are limited to three competing and contrasting conceptions

42. The author most likely refers to the dialectical materialist view of totality as "most challenging" because
    A. few philosophers other than Marx espouse it
    B. it appears to require unprecedented mental capabilities
    C. the insights it offers to a philosopher are overwhelming
    D. it cannot be employed without using the process of abstraction

43. The author includes the example of the chair in order to
    A. point out a complication involved with the dialectical perspective
    B. provide an instance of dialectical abstraction
    C. explain how manufactured objects fit into Marx's view of capitalism
    D. demonstrate that dialectical thinking is impossible

44. The author believes that the dialectical materialist conception of totality
    A. provides insights into the world superior to the ones provided by the atomistic and formalist conceptions
    B. may correctly be found objectionable on certain levels
    C. is impractical when not paired with the concept of abstraction
    D. works best when applied to institutions like capitalism

45. Which of the following would be an example of a dialectical abstraction as detailed in the passage?

    A. A philosopher sees a table as the sum of all the processes that went into producing it.

    B. A philosopher conceives of capital not as a static thing, but as a constantly evolving interaction.

    C. A philosopher studying sexism only looks at developments and changes from the twentieth century.

    D. A philosopher admits that any insights gained are colored by the particular vantage point he or she takes.

46. The primary purpose of the passage is to

    A. argue for the primacy of a particular philosophical ontology

    B. criticize a school of thought as impractical

    C. explain how Marx attempted to study capitalism

    D. attempt to answer a particular objection to a philosophical practice

Questions 47–54 are based on the following passage.

Passage VIII

Biologists use the term "living fossil" to designate a species that maintains many of the features of its ancient ancestors. These species have evidenced very little evolutionary change, indicating not that they are primitive creatures as might be popularly believed, but instead that they are exquisitely suited for their biological and ecological niches and thus have not had any selection pressures to respond to.

The four most celebrated living fossils are the lungfish, the horseshoe crab, the lampshell, and the coelacanth. The horseshoe crab is the relative youngster of the group, belonging to the Jurassic period and having shown little structural changes in its 200-million-year lifespan. The lampshell, a member of the phylum Brachiopoda, is part of an even older lineage, resembling ancestors that lived nearly 400 million years ago.

The oldest members of the living fossil family are the lungfish and the coelacanth, both species that are remarkably similar to their forebears that roamed the Earth almost 425 million years ago. The lungfish, of which there are six surviving species, has the same basic structure and fleshy lobe fins of its progenitor, the sarcopterygian. Of course, the lungfish has long interested biologists not just because of its connections to the distant past but because of the bridge it represents between aquatic species and land dwellers. In fact, the African and South American species of lungfish live part of their lives entirely on land, burrowing into mud and respiring through a tiny breathing hole in their earthy homes. Although the lungfish has remained evolutionarily stable for close to 250 million years, prior to that the species did experience rapid and dynamic evolutionary change. However, by the end of the Permian period, the changes ground to a halt, and the lungfish has persevered happily ever since.

The singular story of the coelacanth stretches all the way from the Silurian period, some 425 million years ago, to the modern day. The coelacanths were well-known from the fossil record and dating technologies placed them in a time when plants were just beginning to encroach on the land. However, biologists thought the species went extinct long before the dinosaurs did. Imagine the surprise when in 1938 a South American trawler captured a strange-looking fish, some five feet in length and a pale blue and silver in color. By an astounding coincidence, the captain of the boat had a relationship with the curator of the East London Museum and had made a habit of sending any interesting finds along to her. Upon seeing this strange specimen, the curator contacted a leading ichthyologist, who, after examining the creature, said he "would not have been more surprised if I had seen a dinosaur walking down the street." But despite all protestations of common sense and amid allegations of forgery and fakery, upon further study, the creature was indubitably a coelacanth. Since that day, explorers have found many more members of the species and have even turned up a second species in the Indian Ocean.

47. The primary purpose of the passage is to
    A. explain how living fossils can remain unchanged by evolution
    B. describe a dilemma facing evolutionary biologists
    C. detail the interesting story of the coelacanth
    D. provide an overview of a biological category

48. The passage states that describing living fossils as primitive is a misnomer because
    A. living fossils are just as advanced as any other species
    B. the public does not understand how evolution works
    C. living fossils continue to evolve
    D. living fossils no longer respond to natural selection

49. Based on the information in the passage, which of the following orderings, from earliest to most recent, is correct?
    A. Jurassic, Permian, Silurian
    B. Permian, Silurian, Jurassic
    C. Silurian, Permian, Jurassic
    D. Silurian, Jurassic, Permian

50. The author probably mentions the lungfish's early evolutionary changes in order to
    A. clarify the term *living fossil*
    B. show that biologists are divided as to what constitutes a living fossil
    C. indicate that the lungfish might again experience evolutionary change
    D. compare the lungfish to the coelacanth

51. The passage suggests that the author most likely believes
    A. the modern discovery of the coelacanth was somewhat due to luck
    B. the lungfish is a more interesting living fossil than the coelacanth
    C. biologists were wrong to think the coelacanth extinct
    D. the coelacanth also experiences a period of rapid evolutionary change

52. In contrast to the other three living fossils, the horseshoe crab
    A. was alive at the same time the dinosaurs were
    B. has experienced few structural changes
    C. is no longer evolutionarily stable
    D. evolved well after land-dwelling plants did

53. The author most likely mentions allegations of forgery and fakery in order to
    A. underscore how unprecedented the discovery was
    B. indicate that some thought to profit from the discovery
    C. describe the public's reaction to the find
    D. dismiss the concerns of leading biologists of the time

54. Suppose a biologist rejects the classification of coelacanths as living fossils. Which of the following pieces of evidence would be MOST helpful to the biologist's argument?
    A. New dating technologies reveal the coelacanth species is only 300 million years old.
    B. A third species of coelacanth is discovered that differs from the other two known species.
    C. New evidence shows that the coelacanth actually belongs to the same lineage as do rays and skates.
    D. A new species of living fossil is discovered that is even older than the coelacanth.

Questions 55–60 are based on the following passage.

Passage IX

For years, a great many political scientists have been puzzled by what appears to be the most basic of all political questions: why vote? Of course, it's not that voting is an overly troublesome or burdensome activity; commonsense explanations of voting behavior are often borne out through empirical study. People vote in order to express their preferences for a particular candidate or platform, to demonstrate their civic pride, or to involve themselves in the political process. The puzzle lies instead in the actual act of voting, which in many ways conforms to what social scientists term the "free-rider problem." Any social good that spreads both costs and benefits amongst a number of citizens encourages the citizens to attempt to reap the benefits without incurring the costs. Given the almost infinitesimal chance that any one individual's vote would actually affect the outcome of an election and given that the supporters of the winning candidate all share equally in the benefit of that candidate's election, the costs of voting, no matter how minor they may be, appear to make voting an irrational act. Better to stay home on election day and let the others do the heavy lifting, the thinking goes.

But the fact is people do get up on election day and vote. Various theories have been postulated to explain this seeming irrational behavior, but there are three factors that political scientists return to again and again: resources, mobilization, and instrumental motivation.

Resources refer to both material possessions such as money and transportation, and immaterial things such as time and political knowledge. Mobilization refers to the pressures the media, political parties, and other groups can exert on an individual in order to make him or her feel compelled to vote. Instrumental motivation is the extent to which a person believes his or her vote will actually affect the outcome of the election.

Of these three critical factors, resources has received the most scholarly attention. According to a classic view of voting behavior, people vote because they have the time and the money to do so. Some political scientists have even calculated what they call a baseline model of political participation. This model attempts to predict political participation based on an individual's level of education, income, and several other occupational variables. Certain individual traits may affect the final decision, but the theory holds that the level of resources is a better predictor of political behavior than any other factor.

Unfortunately, this model, while achieving some success when applied to actual political behavior, suffers from a serious flaw. The model becomes useless when the voting behaviors of citizens from other countries are compared. The differences in voter turnout across educational levels and income are smaller than the differences found in turnout across various countries. Additionally, countries with higher per capita levels of education and income are not necessarily the countries with the highest voter turnout. Indeed, the United States and Switzerland, two countries that are at the top or near to the top of the list in terms of per capita education level and income have some of the lowest voter turnout numbers.

55. According to the passage, the problem that puzzles political scientists is
   A. what motivates people to vote
   B. why people consider voting an irrational act
   C. what makes people think the benefits of voting outweigh the costs
   D. whether voting is a case of the free-rider dilemma

56. The "thinking" referred to in the last sentence of the first paragraph ("Better to stay home on election day and let the others do the heavy lifting, the thinking goes") would most likely be attributed to
   A. political scientists
   B. free riders
   C. typical voters
   D. political candidates

57. According to the baseline model of political participation, which of the following individuals would be MOST likely to vote?
   A. a lawyer
   B. a Swiss citizen
   C. a US citizen
   D. a homemaker

58. Which of the following does the author indicate is a possible factor in explaining voting behavior?
   I. a large amount of free time
   II. get out the vote drives
   III. a sense of the significance of one's vote
   A. I only
   B. II only
   C. II and III
   D. I, II, and III

59. According to the passage, the baseline model of political participation is
   A. applicable only to isolated cases of voting behavior
   B. an accurate predictor of voting behavior
   C. more useful in countries with lower voter turnout
   D. more useful in countries with higher voter turnout

60. The passage implies that
   A. resources are the key factor in explaining voting behavior
   B. the effects of mobilization and instrumental motivation on voter turnout have been ignored by scholars
   C. no theory of voting behavior will successfully explain voter turnout
   D. explanations of voting behavior involving mobilization have not received the same attention as other explanations

STOP. This is the end of Section 4.

ANSWERS AND EXPLANATIONS

Section 1. Biological and Biochemical Foundations of Living Systems

1. **The correct answer is A.** Increasing H^+ ion concentration should drive the reaction to the left, which causes the production of carbonic acid (choice A). If the reaction continues, the carbonic acid would be converted to carbon dioxide and water. This would eliminate choice B, which suggests that the carbon dioxide levels would decrease. Since the reaction is driving to the left, bicarbonate ion levels should not increase, so choice C can be eliminated. The passage indicates that carbonic anhydrase catalyzes the reaction in both directions, so its activity should be increased when H^+ ion concentration increases.

2. **The correct answer is B.** Increased levels of H_2CO_3 in the plasma should lead to an increased production of carbon dioxide and water. Increased levels of carbon dioxide are the primary trigger for ventilation. If carbon dioxide levels are high, the ventilation rate should increase. The presence of carbonic acid would decrease pH as opposed to increasing pH (suggested by choice C).

3. **The correct answer is C.** This question is simply asking for how carbon dioxide is produced on the cellular level. You should recall your knowledge of the process of cellular respiration. During aerobic respiration, glucose goes through glycolysis, Krebs cycle, and the electron transport chain. During Krebs cycle, carbon dioxide is released. Therefore, carbon dioxide is formed in the cells as a by-product of glucose metabolism. Protein synthesis and nucleic acid metabolism do not produce carbon dioxide as by-products.

4. **The correct answer is C.** This question is about osmotic effects. We are told that the process of dialysis needs to remove excess fluids (water) from the blood. In order to do this, the dialysis fluid must have more solutes and less water than the blood. This would mean that the dialysis fluid must be hypertonic to the blood. Another way to say this is that the blood must be hypotonic (contain less solutes and more water) than the dialysis fluid (choice C). If the patient's blood was isotonic to the dialysis fluid, there would be no net movement of water. If the blood were hypertonic to the dialysis fluid, water would enter the blood.

5. **The correct answer is A.** Increasing the levels of Na^+, K^+, and HCO_3^- ions excreted in the urine should increase the concentration of the urine. As the urine becomes more concentrated, osmotic effects occur, and extra water will be excreted with the urine in an attempt to dilute the urine. This will increase the urine volume (choice A).

6. **The correct answer is B.** The question indicates that the toxins being referred to are small in size. We can assume that they are at a high concentration in the blood as compared to the concentration of the dialysis fluid. Choice A can be eliminated because active transport moves substances from a lower concentration to a higher concentration. In this case, we want to move the toxins from a higher concentration (the blood) to a lower concentration (the dialysis fluid). This would indicate that diffusion (choice B) would be appropriate. Osmosis deals only with the movement of water, which will not help move the toxins out of the blood.

7. **The correct answer is D.** Sex-linked inheritance can be quickly eliminated as males and females seem to be equally affected based on the pedigree. Since autosomal inheritance is obvious, it is necessary to determine if the pattern is characteristic of a dominant or recessive condition. Recessive traits are notorious for "skipping generations" in pedigrees, which means that affected children often come from unaffected parents. To be affected, the individual must be homozygous recessive. The parents do not have the disease, but they are unknowing carriers (heterozygotes), which gives them a 25% chance of having an affected offspring. In dominant autosomal inheritance, the affected individual can be homozygous dominant or heterozygous. This means that in order for a child to have the disease, the child must have inherited at least one mutated allele from his or her parent who also had the disease. The only exception would be if spontaneous mutation occurred. When affected individuals appear in each generation of a pedigree, dominance should be suspected.

8. **The correct answer is C.** TSC1 and TSC2 are the normal alleles. Only mutated versions of these alleles cause tuberous sclerosis, according to the passage. The passage indicates that the gene products of TSC1 and TSC2 are hamartin and tuberin, both of which are tumor suppressors. If an individual were to overexpress TSC1 and TSC2, more of the TSC1 and TSC2 gene products would be produced; so we would suspect that their levels of hamartin and tuberin would be elevated. This should provide extra protection against tumor formation, which is indicated by choice C.

9. **The correct answer is D.** The passage explains that individuals who developed tuberous sclerosis as the result of gonadal mosaicism come from parents who do not have the mutated TSC1 and TSC2 alleles in their somatic cells. Since we already determined that the pattern of inheritance for this condition is autosomal dominant, we know that the affected individual only needs to receive a mutated version of TSC1 or TSC2 from one parent. Since individuals inherit their alleles through the egg and sperm of their parents, it is reasonable to expect that the gonadal mosaicism form of tuberous sclerosis must come from a mutation in the TSC1 or TSC2 gene on one of the parent's gametes. Since gametes are made using the

process of meiosis, it would seem that the mutation occurred during this process, leaving choice D as the best answer.

10. **The correct answer is C.** This question relies on the fact that you have already determined that the normal pattern of inheritance for tuberous sclerosis is autosomal dominant. Since affected individuals could be heterozygous for the mutated versions of TSC1 and TSC2, it would be possible that half their gametes carry the normal alleles while the other half would carry the mutated alleles. Assuming both parents with the disease are heterozygous, a Punnett square would indicate that 25% of the offspring would be homozygous recessive and would not have tuberous sclerosis.

11. **The correct answer is C.** We have already established that tuberous sclerosis is an autosomal condition. The passage explains that individuals with the gonadal mosaicism form of tuberous sclerosis come from parents who do not carry the mutated TSC1 and TSC2 alleles in their somatic cells. However, some of their gametes carry the mutation. Since the somatic cells do not have the mutated alleles, these individuals do not appear to have tuberous sclerosis. If a pedigree were to be constructed, it would show two unaffected parents producing a child with the disease. This would resemble autosomal recessive inheritance where "skipping generations" is typical.

12. **The correct answer is A.** This question is asking about anemia, which has many causes. But anemia is always characterized by either a low erythrocyte count or a low hemoglobin count. The question indicated that tuberous sclerosis often occurs as the result of blood loss, which would indicate that the type of anemia occurring would be characterized by low erythrocyte counts and low hemoglobin counts. Since the function of hemoglobin is to transport oxygen, and the hemoglobin and erythrocyte counts are low, it would be expected that oxygen-carrying capacity would be reduced.

13. **The correct answer is C.** The passage explains that lidocaine is metabolized in the liver and produces two metabolites: monoethylglycinexylidide and glycinexylidide. If we are comparing a person with normal liver function to one with compromised liver function, there will be a difference in how long it takes to clear lidocaine from the system. If the liver function is impaired, it is expected that lidocaine will stay in the plasma longer as it waits to be metabolized by the liver. Therefore, the plasma concentration of lidocaine in the liver-compromised patient should be higher after one hour than in the patient with normal liver function. The faster lidocaine is metabolized by the liver, the faster the metabolites would be expected to enter the plasma and ultimately be excreted by the kidneys. Choice C is correct because it suggests that one of the metabolites of lidocaine, monoethylglycinexylidide, would be processed by the liver and kidneys more quickly in the normal patient as compared to the liver-impaired patient.

14. **The correct answer is B.** This question requires an understanding of resting potentials and action potentials in the neurons. Recall that resting potentials (polarization) of neuronal membranes are maintained due to an unequal balance of ions that allows for the inside of the neuron to be more negative than the outside of the neuron. This is primarily due to the action of Na^+/K^+ pumps, which utilize large amounts of ATP to maintain an unequal balance of ions. In the polarized state, Na^+ is found in high concentrations outside the neuron and K^+ is found in high concentrations inside the neuron. The neuron also contains a variety of negatively charged molecules. In order for a message to be sent, the membrane needs to depolarize. This is characterized by the opening of Na^+ gated channels, which allow Na^+ to flood the inside of the neuron, temporarily (and locally) making that area of the neuron more positive inside than outside. This action potential will propagate the length of the neuron, where it will ultimately coerce the release of neurotransmitters into the synapse. Blockage of the Na^+ channels would essentially keep the neuron in resting potential where Na^+ is restricted to outside the neuron. Blocking Na^+ channels prevents the initiation of the action potential or depolarization of the membrane.

15. **The correct answer is A.** Since lidocaine blocks Na^+ gated channels, we have already established that it prevents the initiation of action potentials in the affected neurons. Normally, as action potentials propagate, they eventually cause the release of neurotransmitters into the synapse. Since action potentials are impaired in lidocaine-treated neurons, we should expect that there will be less neurotransmitters released into the synapse.

16. **The correct answer is C.** The passage indicates that lidocaine is an analgesic (prevents pain) by blocking Na^+ gates channels in neurons. Since glial cells are not neurons, choice D can immediately be eliminated. In order to prevent pain from being processed, the messages must be prevented from entering the central nervous system where interneurons are located. Therefore, sensory neurons must be blocked. If these are blocked, the interneurons do not receive the pain messages and motor neurons will not act on them.

17. **The correct answer is C.** Vasoconstriction means that vessel diameter narrows, restricting blood flow to the area. The question introduces the idea of using novocaine during surgery. Since the drug causes vasoconstriction, this would actually increase blood pressure, eliminating choice A. The best choice is C. Bleeding is likely to occur during surgery, so vasoconstriction should slow the blood flow, which results in less blood loss.

18. **The correct answer is B.** This question relies on your knowledge of the anatomy of the heart and the conducting system of the heart. The sinoatrial node (SA node) is a group of conducting cells located in the right atrium. Recall that the valves of the heart are atrioventricular (AV) and semilunar valves. The barricade that divides

the right and left side of the heart is the septum. The SA node generates electrical signals that control cardiac muscle contractions and serves as the pacemaker for the heart.

19. **The correct answer is D.** It is important to provide controls in experimental designs. Control groups should be treated the same as the treatment groups except for the one variable that is being tested. The control group either receives no treatment or receives a placebo (which is not a form of treatment) to make the subject believe that he or she is receiving a treatment. Choices A, B, and C all suggest that the control group should be treated with one of the two drugs (SNP or L-NAME), which removes them as viable options. In the experiment described in the passage, the control group should not be provided with either drug (SNP or L-NAME), which is indicated by choice D.

20. **The correct answer is A.** To answer this question, you need to analyze the data provided. Looking at the number of embryos surviving, you should notice that all three groups treated with any dosage of L-NAME had decreased survival as compared to the control group. The passage explains that L-NAME is a NOS inhibitor. If the enzyme needed to convert L-arginine to NO does not work, then NO levels will be decreased. The data suggest that a decreased level of NO provided by the L-NAME treatment is detrimental. Further, the higher the dose of L-NAME, the more inhibition of NOS and the less NO provided, led to a dose dependent decrease in survival that eliminates choice C as an option. The passage also explains that SNP is a NO donor, which increases NO levels. According to the data provided for the SNP groups, a small increase in NO (seen in group 2) seems to increase embryo survival. However, as the SNP dose becomes larger (and the higher the level of NO provided), this will lead to decreased survival. The highest rates of survival were seen in the 0.1 μm SNP group, and survival decreased with increased dosage of SNP. This would eliminate choice B since increasing levels of NOS would increase NO levels similar to SNP treatment. The data show that SNP treatment (which increases NO levels) is most detrimental to embryo survival. Choice D directly contradicts this. The best conclusion is that NO is necessary for development, since the data showed that the NO inhibition leads to decreased survival. However, only a certain amount of NO is needed as high levels also lead to decreased rates of embryo survival.

21. **The correct answer is B.** Group 1 was the control group, so there would be no need to further investigate that group. This eliminates choice A. Groups 4 and 6 showed drastic decreases in embryo survival, eliminating choices C and D. However, group 2 (choice B) showed an increase in embryo survival, which would suggest that further research within that dosage would be appropriate.

22. **The correct answer is C.** The question relies on your knowledge of the anatomy of the female reproductive system and the events of fertilization. As a follicle ruptures in the ovaries, the ovum would be released into the oviducts. Sperm should enter

the vagina, moving up the uterus and into the oviducts. Sperm should encounter the ovum in the oviducts where fertilization should occur. This eliminates choices A, B, and D, leaving choice C as the correct choice.

23. **The correct answer is C.** This question also relies on your knowledge of early development. After fertilization, the zygote (a diploid, fertilized egg) begins cleavage, which is rapid mitotic cell division. This results in a solid ball of cells. Eventually, the center of this structure hollows out to form a cavity. This stage of development is the blastocyst stage. Choice A can be eliminated because it suggests that a blastocyst is a solid ball of cells when it really is a hollowed-out structure. Choice B suggests a diploid, fertilized egg, which is actually called a zygote. Choice D suggests that there is a ball of cells that perform meiosis. Since we know the only cells to perform meiosis are the gametes, choice D can be eliminated. Choice C correctly describes the structure of the blastocyst.

24. **The correct answer is B.** The passage explains that SNP is a NO donor, which increases NO levels. Since decreased levels of NO can cause reduced blood flow to the extremities, increasing levels of NO may improve blood flow for a diabetic patient.

25. **The correct answer is D.** This question relies on knowledge of the immune response. Interleukins are cytokines that are secreted during the process of clonal selection in primary immune responses. Since they are not specific toward any one particular antigen, choice A can be eliminated. Interferons are produced as nonspecific defenses against viral infections. Virally infected cells secrete interferons that are detected by neighboring cells. Secretion of interferons gives neighboring cells the chance to increase their immune defenses so that they do not become infected by the virus. Since interferons are nonspecific, their presence would not indicate immunity against a specific virus, which eliminates choice B. The components of the complement system circulate in the plasma and are activated by bacteria that may enter the blood. Activation of the complement system ultimately lyses and kills the bacterial cell. Since the question is asking about a virus, choice C can be eliminated because it deals with bacteria. This leaves choice D as the correct response. The detection of antibodies against the viral antigen would indicate that specific defenses were initiated and that plasma cells were activated to secrete antibodies against the viral antigen that was presented by the vaccine.

26. **The correct answer is B.** While polymerase chain reaction (PCR) is used to amplify copies of target DNA, it would not help to get the viral or bacterial genes of interest into plant cells. This eliminates choice A. Choice C suggests that the genes could be cloned into a bacterial cell and transferred to a plant cell by conjugation. Conjugation is unique to certain species of bacteria and occasionally is seen in fungi, but it does not happen in plants. So choice C is eliminated. Choice D

suggests that the genes of interest should be hybridized to the DNA of the plant. Since hybridization occurs between complementary base pairs, this would suggest that the DNA sequence of the gene of interest and the plant would have to be the same, which is not the case. This leaves choice B as the best option. Bacterial or viral genes can be spliced into plasmids. The plasmids serve as vectors to deliver the gene of interest to a variety of cell types, including plants.

27. **The correct answer is D.** Once activated, most cells in the immune system do not live long. Activated cytotoxic T cells and plasma cells are inactivated once the antigen that they have been designed to fight has been eliminated. The basis of long-term immune system protection is the development of memory T and memory B cells (choice D). These memory cells are produced upon primary exposure to a specific antigen and have the ability to survive for years within the body. Should the same antigen return, memory cells quickly proliferate into cytotoxic T cells and plasma cells to fight the antigen.

28. **The correct answer is B.** All vaccines take time to work (often weeks before full immunity occurs), so waiting for an oral vaccine to pass through the digestive tract (which takes no more than a few hours) is not of major concern. This eliminates choice A. Choice C suggests that inflammation in the digestive tract might be a problem. Since the inflammatory response is expected as one of the nonspecific immune defenses, it is not of major concern. Since two choices have been eliminated, choice D is no longer an option. This leaves choice B as the correct response. Since the plant has been engineered to express proteins unique to the virus or bacterium being vaccinated against, it is possible that these proteins might be damaged in the stomach. Recall that the function of the stomach is to digest proteins by using the enzyme pepsin.

29. **The correct answer is B.** This question requires an understanding of the specific defenses of the immune system. The ultimate goal of the specific defenses is to allow for the production of antibodies from plasma cells and the production of cytotoxic T cells. However, neither of these things can occur without the activation of a helper T cell. In order to activate the helper T cell, macrophages must phagocytize foreign antigens. The fragments of these antigens will be displayed on the surface of the macrophage. This antigen presenting cell will then activate the helper T cell.

30. **The correct answer is C.** IgM antibodies are produced first in response to exposure to a new antigen. Later, IgG antibodies will be produced.

31. **The correct answer is C.** Based on the data presented, more of the knockout mice tested positive for the virus than the wild type mice. Since the knockout mice had the new interleukin gene disrupted, they would not produce this new interleukin, which could be the reason that most of the knockout mice tested positive for the virus.

32. **The correct answer is B.** If wild type mice were provided with supplemental inter-leukin X and tested negative for HCV, it is possible that this could be attributed to the presence of interleukin X.

33. **The correct answer is A.** The polymerase chain reaction works by using primers specific to a target sequence. In the presence of that sequence, the primers bind and the target sequence is copied. After multiple cycles, many copies of the target gene are present and can be detected. In the absence of that sequence, the primers do not bind and nothing will be amplified.

34. **The correct answer is A.** The question specifically noted that we were looking for something that was part of the innate set of immune defenses. Of the choices provided, interferons are the only option that would be typical in viral infection.

35. **The correct answer is B.** Because this is an RNA virus that must produce additional RNA viruses, the enzyme's RNA polymerase would be the logical target given that it copies RNA. Reverse transcriptase is unique to retroviruses, and DNA polymerase and DNA gyrase would be used for DNA replication.

36. **The correct answer is C.** Of the choices provided, C is the most plausible. Increased expression of receptors for the new interleukin could lead to a higher level of interleukin activity in the cells. If this interleukin is effective against viral infection, increased activity might lead to better protection.

37. **The correct answer is A.** In positive feedback loops, a stimulus is amplified in the feedback loop. In this case, if the stimulus is the production of an autoinducer, a positive feedback loop would stimulate the production of more autoinducer. This is in contrast to negative feedback loops where the response in the feedback loop is the opposite of the stimulus.

38. **The correct answer is A.** If bacteria can coordinate their efforts to express certain genes, they are more likely to impact their host as compared to if a single cell were to express a gene product on its own. For example, if bacteria were to express a virulence factor, such as a toxin, the impact of that from a single cell would be minimal on the host. However, if the entire population expressed that toxin in a coordinated manner, the impact would be much greater on the host.

39. **The correct answer is B.** As the population of bacteria decreases, and there is less likelihood of a quorum, there is less accumulation of autoinducers within the population. As the population increases, autoinducer expression should increase as well.

40. **The correct answer is A.** The advantage of biofilm formation is that it provides a direct and strong attachment to its host. Biofilms are notoriously difficult to eradicate, and the bacteria within them are provided protection against many variables, sometimes including antibiotics.

41. **The correct answer is A.** This question relies on your knowledge of the structure of organic molecules. The N-AHLs in this question should be recognized as some derivative of an amino acid. Given that information, the most likely way to alter them would be by altering their R group side chains.

42. **The correct answer is D.** Antibiotics must target structures that are unique to prokaryotic cells. Of the choices listed, the nucleus is a structure lacking in prokaryotic cells and therefore could not serve as a target for antibiotics.

43. **The correct answer is C.** The passage indicates that aquaporins are membrane proteins that allow for the exit of water from the cell. Since no other information is given, we should not assume anything else. Choice A suggests that inhibiting aquaporin activity would decrease ion efflux from the cell. Since the passage indicates that aquaporins allow water to leave the cell following the ion efflux, this choice is not appropriate. Choice B indicates that inhibiting aquaporin activity would increase the osmotic gradient across the membrane. Since the passage only tells us that aquaporins influence water movement, this choice can be eliminated. A drug that blocks the activity of aquaporins would prevent water from leaving the cell. If water cannot leave the cell through aquaporins, then there should not be an increase of water loss, as indicated by choice D. The only reasonable explanation is choice C. A decrease in aquaporin activity should mean that less water leaves the cell, so the volume of the cell should not decrease. This means that the apoptotic volume decrease (AVD) should be reduced or decreased.

44. **The correct answer is B.** In order to support the idea that aquaporins are a critical part of the water loss associated with the AVD, it would be necessary to show that water loss does not occur when the aquaporins are inhibited, that water loss is slowed when aquaporins are underexpressed, or that water loss occurs at an accelerated rate when aquaporins are overexpressed. Choice A introduces a cell that overexpresses aquaporins. We would expect that cell to lose more water as a result (increasing the AVD), yet the choice suggests there would be no change in the AVD. A cell that does not express aquaporins at all (choice C) should be unable to lose water so that the AVD would be decreased yet this choice suggests that under these conditions the AVD would be increased. Choice D suggests that a mutated aquaporin gene should cause no changes related to the rate of apoptosis. A mutation in the gene should cause some change to the aquaporins. Of the choices provided, only choice B links an appropriate change in the AVD to aquaporins. If the aquaporins are underexpressed, less water should leave the cell, which would decrease the AVD.

45. **The correct answer is A.** This question relies on your knowledge of membrane potentials. The passage describes that continued depolarization is needed to initiate the AVD. In membrane depolarization, the most critical event is that Na^+ must enter the cell through membrane channels. The Na^+/K^+ pump is used to maintain

membrane polarity and helps restrict Na$^+$ to the outside of the cell and K$^+$ to the inside of the cell. If the pump were to be inhibited, Na$^+$ could enter the cell (and K$^+$ could leave) to cause depolarization as indicated by choice A. Choice B suggests that inhibiting Na$^+$ channels would allow for depolarization of the membrane. However, Na$^+$ channels are required for depolarization. Inhibition of K$^+$ channels as indicated by choice C would not be appropriate either as K$^+$ must leave the cell as a result of depolarization. Choice D is a distractor since Cl$^-$ channels would not be directly related to depolarization.

46. **The correct answer is D.** In order to answer this question, you need to be familiar with electron transport systems that occur within the mitochondrial membranes. Cytochrome c is a component of electron transport systems. If it is released from the membrane, we would expect that electron transport systems would be affected as indicated by choice D. The other choices listed (glycolysis, fermentation, and Krebs cycle) do not rely on electron transport systems; therefore, cytochrome c would not be involved with their function.

47. **The correct answer is C.** A familiarity with eukaryotic cell structures and organelles is needed to answer this question. The organelles that normally contain digestive enzymes are the lysosomes (choice C), which makes them the most likely candidate for being involved with apoptosis. Each of the other choices listed does not deal with destruction of cellular components. The endoplasmic reticulum has two sides—rough and smooth. The rough endoplasmic reticulum is involved with protein production and modification, while the smooth endoplasmic reticulum is involved with lipid synthesis. The Golgi complex sorts and routes contents from the endoplasmic reticulum. Mitochondria are involved with aerobic cellular respiration and the production of adenosine triphosphate (ATP).

48. **The correct answer is C.** This question relies on a knowledge of osmosis and toxicity. In osmosis, water always crosses the membrane from the side that has more water to the side that has less. If the solution outside the cell were isotonic, as suggested by choice A, the solutions and water levels would be equal on both sides of the membrane. This would lead to no net movement of water. Choice B indicates that the solution outside the cell is hypotonic. Hypotonic solutions have more water than what they are being compared to. If the cell were in a hypotonic solution, water would enter the cell, which would be the opposite of what is needed for the AVD. Choice D suggests that the ion efflux creates a situation that makes active transport of water likely. Since osmosis is a form of passive transport, choice D is eliminated. Choice C is the only reasonable choice. If the solution outside the cell is hypertonic, it has less water (and more solute due to the ion efflux) than the inside of the cell. This would lead to water leaving the cell, which is needed for the AVD.

49. **The correct answer is C.** Restriction enzymes are known to cut DNA at specific recognition sequences and are valuable tools for excising genes to be transferred

from one source to another. Reverse transcriptase is used to copy RNA to DNA. Viral vectors can carry DNA of interest into other cells, but they are not used to remove genes from an organism. Polymerase chain reaction (PCR) is used to produce multiple copies of a target DNA sequence.

50. **The correct answer is A.** A series of several genes under the control of a single promoter is most similar to the inducible operon system in bacteria. Okazaki fragments are produced during semiconservative replication on the lagging strand of DNA. Strands of DNA that are hybridized are complementary to each other. A vector is used to carry DNA from one source into another.

51. **The correct answer is C.** Bacterial ribosomes are in fact different from eukaryotic ribosomes. However, the genetic code is universal so there should be no problem translating the proteins. When eukaryotic DNA is introduced to bacterial cells, it is contained in a vector such as a plasmid that is a normal component of many bacterial cells. We know that eukaryotic genes contain introns and prokaryotic genes do not. If a eukaryotic gene is placed in a prokaryotic cell, the introns cannot be removed and the mRNA produced will contain introns. When translated, the intended protein will not be produced.

52. **The correct answer is A.** This question is asking which of the types of tissue listed are epithelial. Skeletal muscle is muscular tissue, adipose tissue is connective tissue, and bone is connective tissue. Epidermal tissue is made of stratified squamous epithelial tissue.

53. **The correct answer is B.** Vaccines are designed to work by stimulating the primary immune response of the recipient. This requires the immune system to recognize an antigen and to mount a specific immune response. Ultimately, this leads to the production of memory cells that can survive for long periods of time. When the system is challenged by the actual antigen, different types of memory cells can quickly proliferate into plasma cells and cytotoxic T cells in order to destroy the antigen.

54. **The correct answer is C.** Genetically modified organisms contain one or more additional genes as compared to their non-GM organism equivalents.

55. **The correct answer is C.** Blood is a fluid made up of liquid plasma (55%), the primary component of which is water, and floating cells (45%). The plasma is richly endowed with dissolved proteins, lipids, and carbohydrates.

56. **The correct answer is A.** This problem can be solved through knowledge of each of the various hormones given in the four options. Antidiuretic hormone maintains control of water balance in the human body by stimulating increased water reabsorption by the kidneys. Luteinizing hormone stimulates secretion of sex hormones by ovaries and testes. Adrenocorticotropic hormone stimulates the adrenal glands. Growth hormone regulates a wide variety of activities involved in growth and metabolism.

57. **The correct answer is B.** The pancreas is the source for two hormones: insulin and glucagon. Among its principal effects, insulin stimulates glycogen formation and storage, stimulates carbohydrate oxidation, and inhibits gluconeogenesis. All of these effects are described in choices A, C, and D. The other hormone, glucagon, stimulates conversion of glycogen into glucose. So choice B is the correct answer.

58. **The correct answer is A.** The superior vena cava is the vein that carries deoxygenated blood from the upper half of the body to the heart into its right atrium. The aorta is the largest and longest of the arteries of the human body that transports oxygenated blood directly from the left ventricle to all other organs and tissues in the body. The hepatic portal vein is the major vein that transports blood from the digestive organs into the liver. The carotid artery is one of two types of arteries (the other being vertebral) that feed blood from the heart and into the head/brain area.

59. **The correct answer is C.** Pulmonary gas exchange is always based on simple diffusion. Diffusion allows for the movement of a substance from an area of high concentration of the substance to an area of low concentration of the substance. Depending on the concentrations, oxygen and carbon dioxide will move in variable directions. Choices A, B, and D indicate that the movement of gases always occurs in a fixed direction, which is incorrect.

60. **The correct answer is C.** Prokaryotic cells lack membrane-bound organelles including a nucleus. Their DNA is circular and does not exist as linear chromosomes. Prokaryotic cells can have a cell wall, but it is typically made of peptidoglycan. The only item on this list that is common between prokaryotic and eukaryotic cells is that they both contain ribosomes needed for protein synthesis within the cell.

61. **The correct answer is A.** This question relies on your knowledge of nutrient breakdown through the digestive system. In the stomach, the primary activity is protein digestion. The enzyme pepsin is activated by the acidity of the stomach. If the stomach pH were to be increased, there may not be enough acid to activate pepsin. This would mean that proteins would not be digested in the stomach. However, the pancreas produces proteinases that can work on protein digestion in the small intestine.

62. **The correct answer is C.** The four major tissue types are listed as choices. Nervous tissue is unique in its communication abilities. Muscular tissue is characterized by bundles of cells with the ability to contract. Epithelial tissue is characterized by sheets or layers of cells that connect to underlying tissues via a sticky basement membrane. Only connective tissues are characterized by cells scattered in a nonliving matrix that often contains fibers such as collagen.

63. **The correct answer is C.** The primary difference between aerobic and anaerobic cellular respiration is the amount of ATP generated. Anaerobic respiration generates 2 ATP per molecule of glucose, while aerobic cellular respiration generates about 36 ATP per glucose molecule.

64. **The correct answer is C.** This problem requires a Punnett square to be performed for each generation. For the first generation, the Punnett square for the genetic cross of TT × tt or:

	T	T
t	Tt	Tt
t	Tt	Tt

In the first generation, the T and t gametes unite to produce individuals with a Tt (heterozygous) genotype. In the second generation, the Punnett square is conducted for the genetic cross of Tt × Tt or:

	T	t
T	TT	Tt
t	Tt	tt

The phenotypic results from this cross are that three of the four pea plants will be tall (TT, Tt, and Tt) and one of the four is short (tt). Thus, the phenotypic ratio of dominant to recessive pea plants is 3:1, given by choice C.

65. **The correct answer is C.** Steroid hormones exert their effects by entering into cells and binding with a receptor in the cytoplasm. The hormone-receptor complex then enters the nucleus where it acts to alter gene expression in the cell. Since the question is asking about nonsteroid, or peptide, hormones, choices A and B can be eliminated. Choice D can also be eliminated as this is not a plausible explanation. Nonsteroid hormones act as first messengers binding to their receptors on the cell membrane. The hormone itself does not enter the cell. The binding of the first messenger to the receptor causes a series of reactions in the cell that ultimately activate second messengers, such as cAMP.

Section 2. Chemical and Physical Foundations of Biological Systems

1. **The correct answer is A.** As the frog follows the parabolic trajectory, the horizontal component of its velocity, which can be calculated by $v_{i,x} = v_i \cos \theta_i$, is positive and remains constant throughout the entire trajectory. Based on this information, one can readily exclude choices B and C as possible answers. The vertical component of velocity begins with its maximum (positive) value at the origin, calculated by $v_{i,y} = v_i \sin \theta_i$, and then follows according to the equation:

   $$v_{f,y} = v_i (\sin \theta) - g \, \Delta t$$

   Thus, at $\Delta t = 0$, the vertical component of velocity of the frog is at its positive maximum value, which decreases until it reaches zero as the frog reaches the maximum altitude or the highest point of its trajectory. As the frog continues past the point of its maximum altitude, the vertical component of velocity begins to increase, but, because the frog is now moving downward, it is negative. The negative values are indicated by the graph moving linearly under the positive x-axis. When the frog lands, the magnitude of the vertical component of velocity is equal to its value at launch but its direction is opposite to that of its launch. The pair of graphs that best represents both components of velocity in projectile motion is choice A.

2. **The correct answer is B.** The energy stored in a capacitor is given by the formula:

   $$E = \tfrac{1}{2} CV^2 = \tfrac{1}{2} (30 \times 10^{-6})(6 \times 10^3 \, V)^2 = 540 \, J$$

3. **The correct answer is D.** The endpoints occur when 1 and 2 equivalents of base have been added. According to the graph, these would be at pH 6 and pH 12.

4. **The correct answer is B.** At pH 2, the amount of H^+ ions in solutions is plentiful. Therefore, both the carboxylic acid and the amino groups are protonated.

5. **The correct answer is B.** Above a pH of 2.4, the carboxylic acid is in the carboxylate form. The amino group is protonated below a pH of 9.8. The zwitterion will exist between pH 2.4 and pH 9.8, making a pH of 6 the correct answer.

6. **The correct answer is B.** A titration is a slow process where titrant is added drop by drop until the endpoint is reached. However, knowing where the steep slope is, one can add more base to begin with and then slow down as the endpoint is approached. Near the endpoint, the slope increases sharply in this area, so smaller increments are needed.

7. **The correct answer is B.** The concentration of the base is twice that of the glycine, so half as much volume is needed to reach the first endpoint. A 50.0-mL sample of 0.050 M glycine will require 25.0 mL of 0.10 M NaOH to reach the first endpoint.

8. **The correct answer is B.** Because the person is walking at a steady pace away from the motion sensor, the velocity is constant. For each increment of time,

the corresponding slope (rise over run) that is the velocity is equal in value throughout the entire activity. Thus, the graph that best illustrates this activity is choice B.

9. **The correct answer is C.** Because the person is walking at a steady pace away from the motion sensor, the velocity is constant. As noted from the previous problem, the graph on a velocity versus time graph is a horizontal line at a nonzero positive value, determined by magnitude of the person's pace. Acceleration, which can be determined by the time rate of change of velocity over time, is zero, because the velocity is constant. This graph is represented by choice C.

10. **The correct answer is C.** In this activity, the person starts at some distance (3 m) away from the motion sensor, which means the graph would have to start at a positive, nonzero value of distance. This readily eliminates choices A and D as possible answers. Since the person is walking toward the motion sensor, the student is walking toward the origin, represented by choice C.

11. **The correct answer is B.** Activity 1 starts with the person standing directly in front of the motion sensor and then walking away from the sensor slowly. This translates into a positively increasing graph (because the person is walking away from the sensor) with a small slope (because the person is walking slowly). The person then stands still, which means the distance remains the same (horizontal line) over that segment. In the final segment, the person walks away, which reveals a graph similar to the first segment appended to the horizontal graph. This is represented by choice B.

12. **The correct answer is D.** In Activity 2, the person starts by standing still (a horizontal line on a distance versus time graph) in front of the motion sensor. The person then walks away from the sensor quickly, described by a positively increasing graph because the person is walking away from the sensor and with a steep slope because the person is walking quickly. In the final segment, the person continues to walk away, again yielding a positively increasing graph but with a smaller slope because the person is walking as opposed to moving quickly. This is represented by the graph in choice D.

13. **The correct answer is C.** In Activity 3, the person starts from a distance of 3 meters and walks toward the motion sensor quickly. Because the person walks toward the motion sensor, the velocity will be negative and represented by a horizontal line for that segment because the person is walking at a steady pace. Because the person moves quickly, the magnitude of the velocity will be greater than if the person was walking slowly. At this point, choices C and D would both be acceptable choices. The person then stands still, which means the velocity is zero and will be zero throughout the entire segment. The person then walks away from the sensor quickly, which is described by a horizontal line of the same magnitude as the first segment but positive because the person is walking away from the motion sensor. The correct answer is choice C.

14. **The correct answer is D.** In Activity 4, the person starts from a distance of 3 meters and walks toward the motion sensor quickly. Because the person walks toward the motion sensor, the velocity will be negative and represented by a horizontal line for that segment because the person is walking at a steady pace. Because the person moves quickly, the magnitude of the velocity will be greater than if the person was walking slowly. The person then walks toward the sensor slowly, which is described by a horizontal line of smaller magnitude than the first segment but still negative because the person is walking toward the motion sensor. In the final segment, the person stands still, resulting in a zero velocity (horizontal line along the x-axis). The correct answer is choice D.

15. **The correct answer is C.** The aqueous phase most effective for providing a pure product would be 1 M sodium hydroxide. The TLC analysis clearly indicates the presence of benzoic acid in the crude reaction mixture. The challenge becomes how to separate benzoic acid from the desired ester using aqueous extraction alone. By using sodium hydroxide in the aqueous phase, benzoic acid is deprotonated to form benzoate, which is soluble in water, as shown. The desired ester lacks the acidic proton and is therefore unaffected by base.

organic soluble   aqueous soluble

16. **The correct answer is B.** The first task is to determine the limiting reagent, which is the alcohol (as shown):

Substance	MW (g/mol)	d (g/mL)	Amt added	mmol
Benzoic acid (**1**)	122	–	1.58 g	13.0
Thionyl chloride	119	1.631	1.04 mL	14.3
(S)-2-methyl-1-butanol (**2**)	88.2	0.819	1.19 mL	11.1
Dichloromethane	84.9	1.325	20 mL	(solvent)

Therefore, the theoretical yield for the product would be 11.1 mmol × 192 g/mol = 2.13 g. The isolated (purified) yield is 1.49 g (according to the experimental), meaning the actual yield is 1.49 g/2.13 g = 70% of theory.

17. **The correct answer is B.** The defining characteristic of the product in the IR spectrum is the carbonyl stretch, which should appear about 1700 cm^{-1}. Spectrum B is the only one that exhibits this band in the IR. Spectrum A shows a stretch at 2200 cm^{-1}, which indicates a nitrile; Spectrum C shows a stretch at 3300 cm^{-1}, which is consistent with an alcohol; and Spectrum D contains no diagnostic peaks aside from C-H and C-C stretches.

18. **The correct answer is A.** The rate would increase. The second reaction involves the Ad_N reaction between an alcohol and an acyl chloride, as shown here:

Since the subsequent reactions (loss of chloride & proton transfer) are rapid, this is the rate-limiting step. Therefore, the rate law for this reaction would be:

$$\text{rate} = k[\text{BzCl}][\text{ROH}]$$

Increasing the concentration of alcohol (ROH) would then increase the reaction rate.

19. **The correct answer is C.** The reaction between an alcohol and a carboxylic acid is very slow. The formation of an ester can be catalyzed by a strong acid (such as sulfuric acid or p-toluenesulfonic acid). However, in this particular case, the acid is first converted to a much more reactive acyl chloride using thionyl chloride, as shown:

20. **The correct answer is A.** The spring constant, k, which is a constant unique to an elastic object that describes the amount of force required to stretch or compress the elastic object by a known distance, can be determined from the data displayed in the first table. Plotting the data with the elastic force, F_{el}, on the y-axis and stretching distance, x_{el}, on the x-axis, the spring constant can be found by taking the slope of the graph. Since the data indicate a linear graph, the slope and thus the spring constant can be found by using the endpoints:

$$k = \text{slope} = \frac{\text{rise}}{\text{run}} = \frac{\Delta F_{el}}{\Delta x_{el}} = \frac{5N - 2N}{0.3m - 0.14m} = \frac{3N}{0.16m} = 18.75\frac{N}{m}$$

21. **The correct answer is D.** The work done in pulling back the slingshot is stored as elastic potential energy, which in turn is transferred to kinetic energy of the moving projectile. Applying the work-kinetic energy theorem:

Work = Elastic Potential Energy = Change in Kinetic Energy

$$= \frac{1}{2}kx_{el}^2 = \frac{1}{2}mv_f^2 - \frac{1}{2}mv_o^2$$

$$v_f^2 = \frac{k}{m}x_{el}^2$$

$$v_f = \sqrt{\frac{k}{m}}x_{el}$$

22. **The correct answer is C.** The percent error can be found from the following equation and substituting in the appropriate values:

$$\%\text{Error} = \left[\frac{\text{Predicted Value - Observed Value}}{\text{Predicted Value}}\right] \times 100\%$$

$$= \left[\frac{3.94\text{m} - 2.64\text{m}}{3.94\text{m}}\right] \times 100\% = 32.9\% \approx 33\%$$

23. **The correct answer is D.** The horizontal landing distance, Δx, can be determined from the equation:

$$\Delta x = v_x\, \Delta t$$

From the response to Question 21, the horizontal velocity that the marble leaves the tabletop with is given by:

$$v_f = v_x = \sqrt{\frac{k}{m}x_{el}}$$

The time can be found using the equation for displacement in the y-direction for accelerated motion:

$$\Delta y = \frac{1}{2}g\Delta t^2$$

Solving for Δt yields:

$$\Delta t = \sqrt{\frac{2\Delta y}{g}}$$

Substituting into the expression above for the horizontal landing distance gives:

$$\Delta x = v_x\, \Delta t = \left[\sqrt{\frac{k}{m}x_{el}}\right]\left[\sqrt{\frac{2\Delta y}{g}}\right]$$

24. **The correct answer is A.** The students are being asked to extrapolate from the data points already collected and displayed in the second table. Performing simple linear regression analysis, the graphed data reveal the following graph of a line:

$$y = 88.3x + 0.895$$

Substituting the value of 10 cm or 0.1 m into the regression line for x, the y-value or the observed value the students should expect to see when the slingshot is pulled back to 10 cm is:

$$y = 88.3\,(0.10) + 0.895 = 9.73\,\text{m}$$

25. **The correct answer is A.** Using the expression for the horizontal landing distance as shown in Question 4:

$$\Delta x = v_x\, \Delta t = \left[\sqrt{\frac{k}{m}x_{el}}\right]\left[\sqrt{\frac{2\Delta y}{g}}\right]$$

If the mass of the marble were doubled,

$$\Delta x = v_x \, \Delta t = \left[\sqrt{\frac{k}{2m}} x_{\text{el}} \right] \left[\sqrt{\frac{2\Delta y}{g}} \right]$$

So, in comparison to the original mass of the marble, the horizontal landing distance would decrease by $\sqrt{2}$.

26. **The correct answer is C.** The answer choices are best considered as two sets of two: two boat conformations and two chair conformations. Boat conformations in general are almost always of higher energy owing to the so-called flagpole interactions shown here:

The distinguishing characteristic between the two chair conformations is that one (choice C) places the chlorine substituent in an equatorial attitude, whereas the other (choice D) forces the substituent to occupy an axial position. An equatorial orientation is almost always energetically preferable.

27. **The correct answer is D.** The first part of the Strecker synthesis involves the nucleophilic addition of ammonia onto the carbonyl carbon of the aldehyde, as shown. The aldehyde therefore functions as an electrophile.

28. **The correct answer is C.** In the second part of the Strecker synthesis, a nitrile group is converted to an acid functionality. The two oxygen atoms in the latter are supplied by water, making this a hydrolysis reaction. Oxidation and reduction can be ruled out by examination of the oxidation state of carbon in the reactant (nitrile) and product (acid). In both compounds, the reactive carbon (in blue) has three bonds to an electronegative element—nitrogen in the nitrile and oxygen in the acid. The oxidation state of the blue carbon is +3 in both cases; therefore, no redox chemistry has occurred.

29. **The correct answer is D.** The valine synthesized in the Strecker synthesis is best described as a racemic mixture and optically inactive. The product of this reaction (valine) clearly has a chiral center; therefore, the two achiral responses are invalid. Since the synthesis launches from an achiral material, and no chiral reagents are introduced along the way, the only reasonable outcome is to have a racemic mixture of enantiomers. Note that the chiral center is set in the first part of the synthesis

(attack of cyanide on the imminium intermediate). Since the attack can occur from either face of the imminium with equal probability, we expect to see an exactly 1:1 mixture of enantiomers. Any racemic mixture is optically inactive because for every molecule that rotates light clockwise, there exists an enantiomer, which will rotate light counterclockwise, resulting in no net rotation.

30. **The correct answer is D.** In the presence of sodium hydroxide, the amino acid (3) will become deprotonated and form the aminocarboxylate (i.e., 4), which will be water soluble. The aminonitrile (2), on the other hand, lacks an acidic proton and will remain neutral. Thus, it will be dissolved in the dichloromethane, which the passage indicates is the bottom layer in the separatory funnel.

31. **The correct answer is A.** The best IUPAC name for compound 2 is 2-amino-3-methylbutanenitrile. The nitrile is the higher order functional group, relegating the amine functionality to substituent status. Therefore, the main chain is a butanenitrile (shown in blue). Note that the nitrile carbon is C1 (this is easy to overlook). Attached to the main chain are an amino group at C2 and a methyl group at C3.

32. **The correct answer is C.** This problem can be solved by substituting the results of each scenario into Poiseuille's law and searching for the largest value. Choice A yields an $8\times$ increase in flow. Choice B results in a $1/32\times$ increase in flow. Choice C yields a $32\times$ increase in flow while choice D results in a $1/8\times$ increase in flow.

33. **The correct answer is A.** By definition of the two types of lenses, a concave lens increases the focal length of an image while a convex lens reduces the focal length of an image. Therefore, choices B and C are incorrect and can be immediately excluded. Since myopia results in image formation in front of the retina, the appropriate corrective lens would be a concave lens, which increases the focal length of the image, causing the image to focus past this point and on the retina. Choice A is the correct response. Choice D represents the corrective approach for hyperopia or farsightedness.

34. **The correct answer is D.** The problem can be solved using the radioactive decay equation:

$$A = A_o e^{-\left(\frac{0.693}{T_{1/2}}\right)t}$$

where A is the final radionuclide activity measured at some time, t; A_o is the initial radionuclide activity; $T_{1/2}$ is the radionuclide half-life; and t is the radioactive decay time. Adapting the given information to this equation, A is the unknown, $A_o = 28 \, mCi$, $T_{1/2} = 5.25 \, d = 453{,}600 \, s$, and $t = 7 \, d = 604{,}800 \, s$, which yields the following calculation:

$$A = (28 \, mCi)(0.397) = 11.1 \, mCi$$

35. **The correct answer is C.** Calcium carbonate (marble/chalk) is insoluble in water and will produce the least amount of ions to spread out in solution. This is different from the other three, which are soluble and will have ions spread out in solution. Calcium carbonate will be soluble in acid, however, which is why acid rain can erode marble statues.

36. **The correct answer is D.** Unknown C is soluble in water, which eliminates the calcium carbonate. Unknown C also forms a precipitate with NH_3. This will happen when magnesium sulfate reacts with ammonia according to the reaction:

$$2 \, H_2O \, (l) + 2 \, NH_3 \, (aq) + MgSO_4 \, (aq) \rightarrow Mg(OH)_2 \, (s) + (NH_4)_2SO_4 \, (aq)$$

37. **The correct answer is B.** Unknown A is soluble in water and has negative results for all of the tests except for conductivity, so it must be NaCl.

38. **The correct answer is A.** The endpoint of a titration should best be matched to the pK of the indicator. Because a strong base and weak acid titration will have an endpoint in the basic range, phenolphthalein is better suited for this titration.

39. **The correct answer is A.** If the $pH = 10$, then the pOH is 4 because $pH + pOH = 14$. Given the $pOH = 4$, the $[OH^-]$ is 1×10^{-4} M. When the K_{sp} expression is written for magnesium hydroxide, we get $K_{sp} = [Mg^{2+}][OH^-]^2$. This then becomes $K_{sp} = [x][x]^2 = [x]^3$. $[1 \times 10^{-4}M]^3 = 1 \times 10^{-12}$. This is close to the actual value of 1.6×10^{-12}.

40. **The correct answer is C.** You first need to determine a mathematical relationship for surface tension, which can be derived from the following equation:

$$h = \frac{2T}{\rho g r}$$

Rearranging the equation for T and substituting all given information yields:

$$T = \frac{\rho g r h}{2} = \frac{\left(1{,}000 \, \frac{kg}{m^3}\right)\left(9.8 \, \frac{m}{s^2}\right)(0.0025 \, m)(0.08 \, m)}{2} = 0.98 \, \frac{kg}{s^2} \approx 1.0 \, \frac{N}{m}$$

41. **The correct answer is A.** This problem can be answered by referring to the equation for the height of the dye traveling through capillary action:

$$h = \frac{2T}{\rho g r}$$

Of all of the options presented for consideration, the only one with direct relevance to a variable within the equation is choice A. The weight of the water is reflected by the term ρg, which must be pulled up the stem by the surface tension. The presence of sugar increases the weight of the water to be taken up the stem by capillary action and thus it travels more slowly. At each time interval recorded in the experiment, the dye in beakers 2 and 3 does not travel as high up the stem as the stem placed in beaker 1.

42. **The correct answer is B.** The equation for the line of best fit for the data recorded for beaker 3 is:

$$y = 0.275x - 0.2$$

which is expressed in the form of the equation for a line:

$$y = mx + b$$

where m is the slope of the line. It is the slope that provides the hourly rate of ascension of the dye up the carnation stem.

43. **The correct answer is C.** The equation for the line of best fit for the data recorded for beaker 1 is:

$$y = 0.945x + 0.26$$

or

Height of Dye $= 0.945 \times$ (time) $+ 0.26$

Substituting the value 10 hours for time yields:

Height of Dye $= 0.945 \times 10$ hrs $+ 0.26 = 9.71$ cm

44. **The correct answer is D.** The equation for the line of best fit for the data recorded for beaker 2 is:

$$y = 0.58x - 0.42$$

or

Height of Dye $= 0.58 \times$ (time) $- 0.42$

Substituting the value of 10 cm for the height of dye and solving for time yields:

10 cm $= 0.58 \times$ (time) $- 0.42$

Time $= 17.9$ hours ≈ 18 hours

45. **The correct answer is B.** The property of t-butoxide (versus methoxide) that is the most significant factor in the lower yield of ether is increased steric bulk. While

t-butoxide does have a higher pKa, this should also make it more nucleophilic. However, engaging in S$_N$2 reactivity is sterically more demanding than proton abstraction. Therefore, the bulkier *t*-butoxide forms less ether.

46. **The correct answer is D.** The thermodynamic product is defined as the one that is thermodynamically more stable. In this case, the internal alkene would be more stable, since it is disubstituted versus the monosubstituted terminal alkene. In an E2 paradigm (which is generally irreversible), one must assume that the major product formed the fastest. In the case of methoxide, this is the internal alkene. Therefore, the internal alkene is both the kinetic and thermodynamic product (actually, the norm).

47. **The correct answer is B.** The terminal alkene is the kinetic product; the internal alkene is the thermodynamic product. The thermodynamics of the products have not changed; thus, the internal alkene is still the thermodynamic product. However, with *t*-butoxide the terminal alkene forms the fastest; therefore, it is the kinetic product.

48. **The correct answer is D.** The most reasonable product distribution is 20% ether; 50% terminal alkene; 30% internal alkene. Since the steric bulk of isopropoxide is intermediate between methoxide and *t*-butoxide, it is reasonable to expect the outcome in all cases to be between the bounds of the other two bases. Thus, more ether is formed than with *t*-butoxide, but less than with methoxide. Furthermore, the terminal alkene is still favored, but less strongly than *t*-butoxide.

49. **The correct answer is B.** The most reasonable product distribution is 50% ether; 50% terminal alkene; 0% internal alkene. With 1-chlorohexene, it is mechanistically impossible to access the internal alkene. Therefore, the only viable products are the ether (S$_N$2 product) and the terminal alkene (E2 product).

50. **The correct answer is B.** The wavelength, λ, of light is related to its frequency, f, by the equation:

$$c = f\lambda$$

where c is the speed of light in a vacuum or $3.0 \times 10^8 \frac{m}{s}$. Solving for the frequency yields:

$$f = \frac{c}{\lambda} = \frac{3.0 \times 10^8 \frac{m}{s}}{700 \times 10^{-9}\,m} = 4.0 \times 10^{14}\,Hz$$

51. **The correct answer is C.** The speed of light through a medium, v, is related to its index of refraction, n, by:

$$n = \frac{c}{v} = \frac{\text{speed of light in vacuum}}{\text{speed of light in medium}}$$

The index of refraction of the aqueous humor is given in the passage as $n_{\text{aqueous humor}} = 1.336$.

Substituting into the above equation:

$$v = \frac{c}{n} = \frac{3.0 \times 10^8 \frac{m}{s}}{1.336} = 2.2 \times 10^8 \frac{m}{s}$$

52. **The correct answer is B.** The speed of light through the medium is related to its index of refraction by the equation:

$$n = \frac{c}{v} \text{ or } v = \frac{c}{n}$$

So the speed of light is slowest when the index of refraction is the greatest. Of the possible answer choices, the medium with the greatest index of refraction is the lens with $n = 1.406$. Thus, the speed of light is the slowest as it passes through the lens of the human eye.

53. **The correct answer is D.** The angle of refraction is determined by Snell's law of refraction or:

$$n_1 \sin \theta_1 = n_2 \sin \theta_2$$

From information given in the passage:

$$n_1 = n_{air} = 1.000; \theta_1 = \theta_i = 28°; \text{ and } n_2 = n_{cornea} = 1.376$$

Solving for the unknown θ_2:

$$\sin \theta_2 = \frac{n_1 \sin \theta_1}{n_2} = \frac{(1.000)\sin 28°}{1.376} = \frac{0.469}{1.376} = 0.341$$

$$\theta_2 = \sin^{-1}(0.341) = 19.9° \approx 20°$$

54. **The correct answer is A.** When light refraction is at its greatest, the refraction angle is the smallest, which occurs when the ratio of $\frac{n_1}{n_2}$ is the smallest. Of the four possible combinations, the smallest value for the ratio is given by the air–cornea interface.

55. **The correct answer is A.** The only true statement is choice A. At the beginning of the reaction, the concentration of the reactants is greatest. This will give the greatest instantaneous rate. Choice B is not correct because, as the reaction nears its end, the rate at that point will be less than the average rate.

56. **The correct answer is C.** First the change in molarity is needed. Then this is divided by the time interval. The initial rate $= (0.882 - 0.697)/60 = 0.00308$ M/sec.

57. **The correct answer is B.** Using the equation $\ln([A]_0/[A]_t) = kt$, substitution gives:

$$[\ln(.882 - .697)] / 60$$

58. **The correct answer is B.** The half-life is the time it takes for half of the starting material to react. Starting with 0.882 M, the first half-life would be at 0.441 M, which would take between 180 and 240 sec.

59. **The correct answer is A.** Because the decomposition is first order, the rate $= k$ [H_2O_2].

60. **The correct answer is A.** A catalyst lowers the energy of activation of a reaction by changing the mechanism of the reaction.

61. **The correct answer is D.** Compound 1 has a good leaving group (bromide), and it is treated with a very strong, hindered base (LDA). Because LDA is so sterically hindered, any kind of substitution (S_N1 or S_N2) is out of the question.

Moreover, the generation of a double bond in the product is a tip-off to an elimination reaction. Choosing between an E1 or an E2 reaction, it is important to
recognize that E1 reactions generally occur in systems where a base is either weak
or nonexistent. Since LDA is a very strong base ($pK_a = 36$), an E2 mechanism is the
most reasonable choice.

62. **The correct answer is D.** The major conformer in the (*1S, 4R*)-isomer lacks the
proper orbital alignment. In both isomers, the *t*-butyl group (shown in blue) locks
the cyclohexane into the chair conformer that gives the *t*-butyl group the equatorial position. Recall that for E2 elimination to proceed quickly, an antiperiplanar
relationship must exist between the leaving group (in this case, bromide) and an
adjacent proton, which is dictated by the alignment of the σ^* orbital of the C-Br
bond with the σ orbital of the C-H bond. The antiperiplanar arrangements are
shown below in bold blue. Notice that the (*1R, 4R*)-isomer can achieve the necessary antiperiplanar arrangement, whereas the (*1S, 4R*)-isomer cannot (a C-C bond
in the ring is antiperiplanar to the bromine).

(*1R, 4R*)-Compound 1

(*1S, 4R*)-Compound 1

63. **The correct answer is A.** Since the dimethyl group at C2 prevents elimination from
the left side, there is only one possible elimination product. Furthermore, since
the reaction does not involve the stereochemistry of the *t*-butyl group, the product
should be a single enantiomer (the *R*-isomer). Inasmuch as only one enantiomer
is present, the product should exhibit optical activity.

64. **The correct answer is C.** Ozonolysis has the net effect of cleaving the double bond and putting two carbonyl groups in its place. Choices A and B differ from choices C and D by the total carbon count. Note that the starting material (compound 2) has six carbons in the ring—these six carbons will end up as six carbons in the chain of the dialdehyde (compound 3). Choices A and B only have five chain carbons; therefore, they can be disqualified. The remaining choices (C and D) differ in the stereochemistry at the *t*-butyl group. Ozonolysis will not affect this stereochemistry, as shown:

65. **The correct answer is C.** Bear in mind that the regiochemistry in hydroboration is driven by sterics alone. In this particular case, there is no clear Markovnikov or anti-Markovnikov product (i.e., both product alcohols are similarly substituted). However, there is a difference in the steric interactions involved in the two approaches of the borane molecule to the double bond. If the boron aligns with the carbon at the 12 o'clock position, there is steric hindrance caused by the dimethyl group, as shown. This interaction is absent when the boron aligns with the carbon at the 2 o'clock position. The hydroxy group ends up at the same position that the boron was added. As for the stereochemistry of the *t*-butyl group, it is unaffected by this chemistry.

Section 3. Psychological, Social, and Biological Foundations of Behavior

1. **The correct answer is D.** The "swinging bridge" study showed that in conditions eliciting a stronger adrenaline reaction, participants rated others as more attractive. This result highlights certain environmental factors that can alter the judgment of attractiveness. This phenomenon is called misattribution of arousal.

2. **The correct answer is B.** Broca's area in the left frontal lobe is responsible for language production in the brain. In this example, the individual understands language (written) but is unable to produce speech. Interestingly, patients can often produce language if they sing, and this is a frequent therapy for individuals with damage to Broca's area.

3. **The correct answer is C.** Though Janey worked hard for her degree and is excited about her career, it is her father who provides a job for her rather than having her interview and receive the position through normal channels. If she received a better job based on her own hard work and better grades, the sociological construct would be meritocracy. A social mobility construct would indicate that she had changed from one socioeconomic status (SES) level to another, but in this instance Janey is maintaining her same SES with a career in the same field as her father. This suggests social reinforcement rather than social mobility. Social stratification indicates that different SES levels exist and does not really apply in this case.

4. **The correct answer is A.** The door-in-the-face technique is characterized by an outrageous request followed by a second, more reasonable request. In this example, the outrageous request is the offer of overpriced jewelry. The reasonable request is the offer of less expensive jewelry.

5. **The correct answer is C.** As mobility has increased, residents of a particular area are less likely to retain traditional norms and customs that historically characterized the area. As mobility increases, the population of an area is more likely to change, and this will lead to less uniform culture and the potential loss of local customs and traditions.

6. **The correct answer is C.** The Young-Helmholtz theory of color vision posits that color vision depends on three pigment receptors. Each of these receptors has different spectral sensitivities. Light of a particular wavelength activates the pigment receptors to different degrees, and the pattern of activity represents the perceived color. Ewald Hering proposed the opponent-process theory of color vision. This theory posits that color vision is caused by opposing responses generated by blue and yellow wavelengths and by red or green wavelengths (black and white are also sometimes added).

7. **The correct answer is C.** The photo receptors will all respond to the wavelength of light. However, certain wavelengths will result in increased relative activation compared to others. This relative activation results in the perception of color.

8. **The correct answer is B.** The trichromatic (Young-Helmholtz) theory posits that receptors are stimulated within a range of wavelengths. So while they are preferentially stimulated by certain wavelengths, they respond to many. This is true for both rods and cones. Further, the combination of the three cone pigment receptors creates the perceived color.

9. **The correct answer is D.** A person lacking red- or green-sensitive cone pigment receptors would have red-green color blindness. The photoreceptors' stimulation curves overlap substantially, and the lack of either can be classified as red-green color blindness.

10. **The correct answer is A.** Wavelength stimulates the cone receptors. The combination of stimulation from the wave creates the perception of color. The perception of brightness results from the amplitude of the wave. The intensity of the stimulation increases, but the relative activation of the cone receptors stays relatively the same.

11. **The correct answer is C.** Men are more likely than women to use resource display. Based on the data shown, men are more likely to engage in resource display as a mate retention strategy.

12. **The correct answer is A.** Evolutionary psychology would explain that men are more likely to use resource display because women value financial status as a characteristic in a mate. Evolutionary psychology posits that women are more likely to pursue mates who can provide resources for potential offspring because that indicates that their future offspring will be more likely to survive and pass on the women's genes.

13. **The correct answer is B.** Males select mates based mainly on the youth, attractiveness, and good health of their potential partner. This answer is consistent with males selecting mates that have characteristics indicating higher potential fertility.

14. **The correct answer is D.** A likely potential follow-up investigation would study the correlation between behavior and the financial status and perceived attractiveness of the mates. This would allow for a comparison of retention strategies used, based on previously identified desirable characteristics in male and female populations.

15. **The correct answer is D.** Women are more likely to use indirect means of communicating to competitors that their spouses are "taken." Nonverbal possession signals allow communication without the threat of violence, which may damage health, childbearing ability, and physical well-being (all of which are key attractors to men, according to evolutionary theory). In this instance, public displays of affection are used as a signal to competitors, not as a way to make a partner commit.

16. **The correct answer is D.** Amnesics experience impairment for explicit memory tasks but do not experience impairment for implicit memory tasks compared to

control participants. The amnesics score significantly lower on the explicit memory tasks. However, there is no significant difference in performance on the implicit memory tasks.

17. **The correct answer is B.** Amnesic participants were significantly worse at explicit memory tasks compared to control participants. Further, they were able to complete the implicit memory task for a novel (learned) list of words. This suggests that they are able to encode new information (i.e., learn) but are unable to explicitly recall or retrieve the previously stored information.

18. **The correct answer is A.** Amnesic patients are able to encode and access semantic memory but are still impaired in their ability to retrieve the encoded information. Amnesic patients are able to perform the implicit memory task, and so are able to encode information. However, they are impaired in their ability to retrieve information unless that information is prompted in the implicit task. Further, it is possible that the patients were able to explicitly recall the experience of learning and form an episodic memory. However, the only answer choice that includes episodic memory can be ruled out because semantic memory is necessary for episodic retrieval in Tulving's model.

19. **The correct answer is C.** The hippocampus has been found to be a critical structure in the storage and retrieval of memories. Patients with damage to the hippocampus have impaired memory formation and retrieval.

20. **The correct answer is C.** Memories are stored in various locations throughout the cerebral cortex through a process called long-term potentiation.

21. **The correct answer is C.** Participants were better able to remember which list familiar melodies were from than novel melodies. List recognition was better for familiar melodies than for novel melodies for both studied lists.

22. **The correct answer is A.** Episodic memory is characterized by the ability to identify and consciously re-experience an event that occurred in the past. Procedural, semantic, and implicit memory are characterized as memory of an event without a corresponding knowledge of when it occurred.

23. **The correct answer is B.** Semantic memory is characterized by the ability to recall facts but not remember when an event occurred. In this case, the semantic memory provides the knowledge that the melody is known but is unable to isolate when the melody was heard.

24. **The correct answer is A.** Long-term potentiation has created long-lasting excitatory circuits for the memory trace. Long-term potentiation is the process by which memories are stored and lasting memories are encoded.

25. **The correct answer is D.** The percentage of familiar melodies correctly ascribed to both list 1 and list 2 would decrease. Participants would be unable to ascribe familiar melodies to either list because they would not have a memory of when they heard each melody.

26. **The correct answer is A.** The results show a significant increase in acts of imitative aggression by children who view a film showing aggression being rewarded.

27. **The correct answer is C.** Bandura's research showed that children would imitate aggression when they viewed the aggression rewarded. Learning was not directly tested, and children only needed to view the aggression (reward/punishment) conditions.

28. **The correct answer is B.** The offending child in the example is punished for the child's actions despite the initial aggression. This is consistent with the aggressive-model-punished condition of Bandura's study in which the child is initially aggressive and is later punished for his or her actions.

29. **The correct answer is D.** One major criticism of Bandura's study was that the children were in an artificial environment and displayed aggression toward a toy rather than toward another child (as seen in the film).

30. **The correct answer is A.** Joey watches a friend play a violent video game in which punching small animals results in more points. In this condition, Joey is watching his friend being rewarded for aggressive behavior.

31. **The correct answer is D.** According to the regression lines in the two graphs, in a country with an average fertility rate of six children per woman, a girl has approximately a 22% chance of being enrolled in secondary school and an 80% chance of living on less than $2.00 per day.

32. **The correct answer is B.** Each living child alters the financial resources available to each family member, and frequent childbirth may increase health problems for the woman, which may impede her ability to be financially productive. A higher number of children leads to fewer financial resources per child because income does not necessarily rise with the birth of each child. Fewer financial resources means fewer educational opportunities, particularly for girl children outside of the United States.

33. **The correct answer is D.** The graphs depict only women's fertility, education, and poverty levels. Men's fertility levels are less well known. Even in the context of marriage, many of the world's cultures have less strict sexual rules for men, making men's fertility much more difficult to track.

34. **The correct answer is B.** Attitude shifts within a culture toward acceptance of family planning would be a change in cultural capital.

35. **The correct answer is D.** Education increases human capital; therefore, education about family planning services would be an increase in a society's human capital.

36. **The correct answer is D.** The group at the highest risk is individuals with a schizophrenic identical twin. The data show that the highest incidence rate (60%) is for identical twins. Children whose parents are both schizophrenic are the group with the next highest risk at 37%.

37. **The correct answer is D.** The data show a strong genetic link for the incidence rate of schizophrenia. However, in the case of identical twins (100% genetic match), the incidence rate is only 60%. This suggests that additional environmental influences must also be factors in the development of schizophrenia.

38. **The correct answer is A.** The other answer choices have been associated with schizophrenia in the research literature. Too much GABA (which is an inhibitory neurotransmitter) has not been associated with schizophrenia in the research literature, although too little GABA has been proposed as a possible mechanism.

39. **The correct answer is A.** The most appropriate follow-up study would be to survey identical twins who grew up apart and those who grew up in the same household. This is the best answer because it would allow you to study individuals who are exact genetic matches with each other and also allow you to compare same-household (similar environments) twins to different-household (different environments) twins.

40. **The correct answer is D.** Because a child's genetic code cannot be changed but environmental factors also play a role in the development of schizophrenia, a child with schizophrenic family members should receive extra environmental support to reduce the likelihood of developing schizophrenia. Schizophrenia is not inevitable based on genetic factors. Choice C is not a real possibility because avoiding all stress is not possible. Antipsychotic medications have serious negative side effects, and treatment guidelines do not recommend that they be started prophylactically for schizophrenia.

41. **The correct answer is B.** The length of time a person spends in REM sleep per sleep cycle generally increases as the night progresses. Amplitude becomes larger and frequency slows down as deeper levels of sleep are reached. Further, the length of time a person spends in slow wave sleep decreases as the hours of sleep increase.

42. **The correct answer is A.** Most vivid dreaming occurs during REM sleep. Dreaming can also occur during other stages, but it is typically not as vivid.

43. **The correct answer is D.** Each sleep cycle is approximately 90 minutes in length. The cycle is characterized by the stages.

44. **The correct answer is B.** REM sleep and slow wave sleep are considered to be associated with restorative processes. REM sleep has been found to decrease as one ages and loss of REM sleep has been found to be associated to cognitive dysfunction (particularly memory). The release of growth hormone during slow wave sleep has physiological benefits.

45. **The correct answer is D.** At 10:30 p.m., Jose had just begun to enter stage 2 sleep, which is a much lighter sleep state than the sleep states represented by the other answers. During stage 2 sleep, Jose is much more likely to be awakened by small noises that would not affect him during slow wave sleep (choices B and C) or at the

onset of REM sleep (2 a.m.). While the end of REM sleep can result in easier arousal from sleep, the onset of REM sleep is associated with more difficult sleep arousal.

46. **The correct answer is D.** Sound level decreased for participants in actual groups and for participants in pseudogroups. The data show that as the number of people in actual groups increased and the number of (supposed) people in pseudogroups increased, the sound level decreased.

47. **The correct answer is B.** The decibel level would decrease if the people in pseudogroups believed that there were more people in their groups.

48. **The correct answer is A.** Loss of coordination is characterized by a decrease in productivity due to role/work overlap. The actual groups and the pseudogroups are both affected by social loafing. This is because the actual groups and pseudogroups both believe that there are others working with them. However, only the actual group is affected by loss of coordination. This difference is explained by the lack of a feedback loop, which would indicate the work overlap in the pseudogroups (who are only told there are others working with them) compared to the actual groups (who receive feedback from other group members present).

49. **The correct answer is C.** The difference between the potential productivity and the pseudogroups' productivity can best be explained by social loafing because the difference is the result of *believed* group size. The pseudogroup participants are not aware of any actual participation by any other person. So loss of coordination does not have any impact on pseudogroup results.

50. **The correct answer is A.** The greater the number of people working together to complete a task, the more likely it is that social loafing will occur due to a diffusion of responsibility, resulting in decreased effort.

51. **The correct answer is B.** This statement is consistent with the results in the figure and shows that increases in shallow acting are likely to result in increases in stress.

52. **The correct answer is C.** In the dramaturgical approach an individual is always playing some type of role in all social interactions. Based on the research shown, deep acting will result in less stress.

53. **The correct answer is B.** Cognitive dissonance theory suggests that if you change your beliefs, acting becomes less stressful. The theory states that in low-reward situations, it is less stressful for you to alter your beliefs to match existing situations. In this example, customer service workers engaged in surface acting (e.g., changing facial expressions, smiling at customers) and deep acting (e.g., detailing the benefits of a product, etc.) in order to interact with customers. Because there is little direct reward for showing enthusiasm and engaging customers, more stress will result with surface acting in which inner beliefs are not changed. Conversely, for deep acting, cognitive dissonance would result in a shift in inner beliefs to match deep acting behavior, resulting in less stress compared to that experienced during surface acting.

54. **The correct answer is A.** Self-verification involves making sure that a person chooses the "audience" that verifies his or her self-view and thus reinforces that person's self-identity.

55. **The correct answer is A.** According to the dramaturgical approach, individuals are truly themselves only when they are alone (off-stage). Onstage behavior is characterized by acting, and backstage behavior is still influenced by goal-directed behavior for the audience.

56. **The correct answer is B.** High-social-contact participants under high stress are more likely to become sick than low-social-contact participants.

57. **The correct answer is D.** Both positive events and negative events increase stress. The more social contacts, the more likely that a person will be exposed to a cold or flu, and the higher the stress, the more likely the individual will become sick.

58. **The correct answer is B.** Taking steps to master, tolerate, or reduce stress is referred to as coping.

59. **The correct answer is B.** Light exercise such as taking a morning run is a positive coping mechanism and will likely reduce stress.

60. **The correct answer is C.** The fight-or-flight response is characterized by the activation of the autonomic nervous system.

61. **The correct answer is A.** Students in the majority of the listed US states score below students in the majority of listed countries in terms of math proficiency. More US states are listed at the lower end of the percentage-proficient scale.

62. **The correct answer is C.** Functionalism posits that different parts of society are separate but interrelated. This view of society supports the status quo and attempts to avoid any disruptions to the system.

63. **The correct answer is B.** To a conflict theorist, the data would reflect attempts to reinforce historical inequities between various state and country populations. Conflict theory posits that society is fundamentally in conflict when there is an uneven distribution of resources. Differences in prestige and resources create fundamental power struggles between groups of people.

64. **The correct answer is C.** Secondary production involves the transformation of raw resources into material goods. High-tech manufacturing is an example of secondary production.

65. **The correct answer is D.** As the highest ranked US state, Massachusetts serves as a model for other states in identifying unique skills and teaching methods to improve their own systems of mathematics education. There is no information about gender disparities or about changes in rankings over time, so choices A and B cannot be correct. Choice C does not apply because the Asian countries on the graph are above the mean in mathematically ability.

Section 4. Critical Analysis and Reasoning Skills

1. **The correct answer is C.** Skim to locate mention of three out of four assertions. The underground system (choice A) appears in paragraph 4, purple loosestrife's effect on fish appears in paragraph 6, and its use in American gardens (choice D) appears in paragraph 2. Paragraph 7 says that it is "impervious to burning," making choice C the best answer.

2. **The correct answer is B.** This question indirectly asks you to locate an author's reasons for including a detail. Returning to the passage will help you see that the mention of the St. Lawrence refers to a type of wetland where purple loosestrife does well. The only answer supported by the text is choice B.

3. **The correct answer is C.** All three details are facts about purple loosestrife, but only its ability to cross-pollinate (I) and its easy adaptability (II) are facts that "add to its power of endurance." Since both I and II are correct, the answer is choice C.

4. **The correct answer is C.** The answer appears in paragraph 3: "The same long growing season that makes it so beloved by gardeners makes it a seed-making machine." It is the long growing season (choice C) that gardeners like.

5. **The correct answer is D.** You must infer the answer based on what you have learned about purple loosestrife from the passage. Because it thrives in wetlands and along rivers, either II or III is likely. Although I might in theory be possible, the author does point out, "It has moved steadily westward and is now found in all states but Florida." Since that eliminates I as a choice, the answer must be choice D.

6. **The correct answer is B.** Your choice must weaken the argument that purple loosestrife is best eradicated by digging it up, plowing it under, and reseeding. Choice A would suggest another means of eradication but would not weaken the original argument. Choices C and D do not weaken or strengthen the argument, although both may suggest benefits of the eradication plan. Only choice B throws a monkey wrench in the works: If a new strain of purple loosestrife is growing up where it was once eliminated, then this form of eradication does not really work.

7. **The correct answer is C.** Native American and Chinese drums are mentioned in the first paragraph as examples of drums that accompany soldiers into battle.

8. **The correct answer is D.** A Janissary stop is described as being added to organs and harpsichords, which have a series of stops, or knobs, that adjust tones and add special effects. The only answer that fits the context is choice D.

9. **The correct answer is C.** Haydn and Mozart enter the discussion as examples of classical composers who adopted the forms and characteristics of martial music. This does not mean that Janissary music came from Europe (choice B), and since Haydn and Mozart are musicians, not painters, choice D does not apply.

10. **The correct answer is C.** Skim the passage to find whether examples are given to support each assertion. Looking first at assertion I, you can see that the author

mentions the "Jingling Johnny" as an example of unusual percussion. Since I is a yes, you can immediately eliminate answer choices B and D. The only question remaining is whether the answer is choice A or C, so you must look for examples to support assertion III. The first sentence in paragraph 4 mentions "The Stars and Stripes Forever" as an example of Sousa's beloved marches. Since I and III are both yes responses, your answer must be choice C.

11. **The correct answer is A.** This is a "what-if?" question: What if the author included this particular piece of information? The fact that it refers to the eighteenth century means that it has no relation to the Civil War (choice C), and the use of drums preceded Janissary music (choice D). The best answer is choice A; it would help support the idea that martial music was a key part of the military at that time.

12. **The correct answer is B.** The author compares the Pentagon's expenditure on music to the government's comparatively paltry expenditure on K–12 music education. Although the information is fascinating (choice A), the shock value involved in the comparison makes it most likely to have been included as a critical remark.

13. **The correct answer is C.** Since the whole passage is about military adventures, you should be able to select choice C as the most likely answer without reviewing the passage. The proof is in paragraph 5, where the author refers to "the final campaigns of the Zulu War."

14. **The correct answer is B.** Although Rorke's Drift was a British success story (choice C), the author makes clear that it was a minor success at best and tells how Chelmsford used it to cover up a huge British failure at Isandhlwana.

15. **The correct answer is A.** The author does not seem to think much of the tactics of Frere (choice C), and Wolseley (choice D) is mentioned only in terms of his success after taking over for Chelmsford. In the author's narrative, Chelmsford tried to seize Zululand, but his invasion force was massacred and he was eventually recalled to England. Despite his self-serving propaganda, Chelmsford clearly failed to accomplish his purpose. The best answer is choice A.

16. **The correct answer is D.** King Cetshwayo (choice C) ruled Zululand before he fought the British. After the kingdom was subdivided, a white African mercenary (choice A) ruled one part of it. Later, Dinizulu (choice B) wrested the kingdom from his own brother and ruled briefly. Chelmsford (choice D) never ruled at all.

17. **The correct answer is C.** Your choice must specifically point to a British failure to understand the African culture. Chelmsford's cover-up (I) has nothing to do with the Africans. The three-column advance (II) may have been a tactical error, but it cannot be blamed on a failure to understand Africans. The failure of partition (III), however, indicates that the British did not recognize the divisions among tribal leaders and peoples. Since only III is a yes, the answer is choice C.

18. **The correct answer is D.** To answer this question, you must think about the purpose and aim of the Zulu War. It was not a peasant uprising (choice A) or a war

to eradicate a people (choice B); it was a war designed to topple a leader so as to form a union imposed from outside the region. In that way, it most resembles modern-day Iraq (choice D).

19. **The correct answer is D.** In the last paragraph, the author states that Smith "had inspired many of the changes for which his rival is now known." His rival was Roosevelt, and the implication is that Roosevelt took credit for many ideas that began with Smith. There is no indication that Roosevelt would have done better on a ticket with Smith (choice A), and Smith's background is not a topic of this paragraph (choice C). Contrary to choice B, many of Smith's ideals were those that formed the foundation of the New Deal.

20. **The correct answer is B.** Although choice A may be true, only choice B is alluded to in the passage. New York City, says the author, was "viewed even in the early twentieth century as disconnected from the national character."

21. **The correct answer is D.** Without knowing more about the two rivals, any one of these answers might be possible, but the only one that is supported by the text is choice D. Roosevelt's ambition led to political maneuvering that shut Smith out of the nomination.

22. **The correct answer is B.** The discussion of nativism shows that Smith was not a credible candidate to many because of his Catholic immigrant background. It has nothing to do with his eligibility (choice A); it has to do with the bigotry of the electorate.

23. **The correct answer is D.** Either choice A or choice B might be true, but neither is supported by the text. Davis was chosen as a "compromise candidate" when the delegates failed to choose between Smith and McAdoo.

24. **The correct answer is B.** The author goes into detail about Smith's many successes in the state of New York, from his work as Speaker of the Assembly to his many years as governor. Choice A does not support the claim that he was successful, and choice C actually belies the claim. The list of names mentioned in choice D does not exist in the passage.

25. **The correct answer is A.** Smith was a progressive born of immigrant parents, and he supported both civil liberties and unions as well as "those he saw as most in need of government's assistance." Of the answers given, only choice A is likely.

26. **The correct answer is D.** Hunting and habitat destruction are the only reasons mentioned for the depopulation of elk prior to the twentieth century.

27. **The correct answer is D.** According to the passage, in 1913, 50 elk were moved from Yellowstone to Pennsylvania. Two years later, 95 more were moved. The total shipped in those years comes to 145.

28. **The correct answer is D.** "At present," says the passage, "new herds are established in Arkansas, Kentucky, Michigan, and Wisconsin in addition to Pennsylvania." There is talk of moving herds to Tennessee (choice A) and the Adirondacks (choice C)

in the future. Georgia (choice B) is mentioned only as the original southernmost range of eastern elk; it is not a place where they might be seen today.

29. **The correct answer is C.** A list of states accompanies assertion I, and a list of animal species accompanies assertion II. Since both I and II are supported by examples, the answer is choice C.

30. **The correct answer is B.** As the passage states clearly, "All of the eastern subspecies are now extinct." The reintroduced subspecies is the western subspecies, the one found in Yellowstone. It is a different subspecies from the original Pennsylvania elk.

31. **The correct answer is D.** Your answer must directly support the contention that elk repopulation is carefully monitored. Choices A and C have nothing to do with repopulation; they deal with animals in confined conditions. Choice B deals with wild elk but not with monitoring of the population. Choice D shows an example of monitoring that is taking place today.

32. **The correct answer is C.** The claim is that elk reintroduction benefits other species. Your answer must contradict this contention. Choice A shows a clear benefit to other populations, so it does not contradict the claim. Choice B shows a change in a species that does not live where elk live. Choice D does not refer to other species at all. Only choice C indicates a possible problem; the fact that deer are migrating northward may mean that elk are encroaching on their habitats.

33. **The correct answer is A.** Spooner was known for his transpositions, of which "You have deliberately tasted two worms" (wasted two terms) is an example. Although *transposition* has a variety of possible meanings, here it refers specifically to the exchange of letters or word parts.

34. **The correct answer is C.** The final paragraph discusses two forms of metathesis that derive from the butchers' trade. One is *louchébem* (II), and the other is *rechtub klat*. Since only II is correct, the answer is choice C.

35. **The correct answer is D.** Verlan and other backslang (I) are word games and therefore purposeful, not accidental. The examples of accidental metathesis include the change between Latin originals and Spanish derivatives (II) and mispronunciations or skewed pronunciations of English words (III). Since II and III are correct, the answer is choice D.

36. **The correct answer is D.** Although the origin of Pig Latin appears to be unknown, the author refers to its use in the prisoner-of-war camps of World War II and Vietnam. The implication is that it was used to communicate between prisoners in a language their captors could not understand.

37. **The correct answer is C.** If most Spoonerisms are apocryphal, or fictional, that would not be proved by a list of attributed transpositions (choice A), which would simply seem to support their authenticity. Examples of modern-day transpositions (choice B) would do nothing to support or deny the authenticity of Spoonerisms, and Spooner's letters (choice D) would not help because his transpositions,

if they existed, were oral, not written. Interviews with people who knew Spooner (choice C) would be the best way to settle the issue one way or the other.

38. **The correct answer is B.** Saying *cause* instead of *because* (III) is an example of *aphaeresis*, the loss of the initial part of a word. The other two examples show transpositions of phonemes that are accidental. Since I and II are correct, the answer is choice B.

39. **The correct answer is B.** Verlan transposes the phonemes in syllables, often changing the spelling to match the revised word construction. Since *critique* is pronounced /krih-teek/, reversing those phonemes would give you a word pronounced /teek-krih/. The most likely spelling for this is shown in choice B.

40. **The correct answer is C.** Compare what you know about Pig Latin to what you know about metathesis. Pig Latin, like other metathesis, does transpose phonemes, so choice A is incorrect. Metathesis may be accidental or purposeful, so choice B is incorrect. There is no indication that the definition of metathesis includes the rule that such words must add to the language, so choice D does not work. Pig Latin involves more than the reversal of phonemes that marks metathesis; it also involves the addition of the "ay" syllable. The best answer is choice C.

41. **The correct answer is C.** This question involves your understanding of supporting details and evidence. The answer is found at the beginning of the passage, where the author details the three conceptions of totality. Here, the author states that the first two views are "contrasting" and that the third view is "not simply . . . the sum of its parts as atomists believe or . . . something independent of its parts." Thus, all three views are incompatible with each other, and choice C is the correct answer. There is no evidence that the views have evolved from each other (choice A). The materialist view is one of the conceptions of totality, and it has helped philosophers grasp connections, so choice B cannot be correct. Be careful of choice D; the passage states that philosophers "recognize" three different view, but that doesn't mean there are only three views.

42. **The correct answer is B.** This question asks you to assess evidence. What supporting evidence does the author give to back the claim that this view is "challenging"? The answer lies at the end of the third paragraph, where the author states that the high number of connections and relationships make the view "overwhelming" to even the brightest philosophers. This idea is what choice B expresses. It is not clear from the passage how many philosophers espouse this view (choice A), and the author doesn't say whether that makes the viewpoint challenging. Choice C is wrong because the author says the number of things a philosopher must consider is overwhelming, not the insights. The author says that Marxist philosophers use abstraction (choice D) but never states that it is necessary to the dialectical viewpoint.

43. **The correct answer is A.** This question depends on your ability to analyze an argument. The author uses the chair in the third paragraph as part of his discussion on the critics' objections to a dialectical conception of totality. This is precisely what choice A states. The author has not yet discussed abstraction (choice B) or capitalism (choice C). Choice D is too strong; the author doesn't say dialectical thinking is impossible, just difficult.

44. **The correct answer is B.** In order to answer this question you need to distinguish among fact, opinion, and unsupported assertions. Look in the passage for the author's opinion or belief about the dialectical materialist viewpoint. At no point does the author indicate it leads to superior insights (choice A). *Critics* of the view state that it is impractical to use, but the author doesn't state that is what *he* believes (choice C). And there is no indication that the author thinks it's best used for the study of institutions (choice D). That leaves choice B, which is supported when the author writes that criticisms of dialectical materialism are "somewhat justified." This gives an indication of the author's belief about his subject matter.

45. **The correct answer is C.** This question asks you to draw conclusions. Using the information in the passage, you must conclude which answer choice reflects a process of abstraction. The author states that abstraction allows the investigator to "draw boundaries" around an object or idea studied. One possible abstraction involves "time scale." In choice C, the philosopher puts a temporal boundary around the idea studied. Choices A and B are examples of dialectical thinking but not abstractions. Choice D simply indicates a philosopher is aware of his or her biases, but there are no abstractions made.

46. **The correct answer is D.** To answer this question you'll need to look for the main idea. Choice A is not correct because the author does not say that the dialectical viewpoint is better than the other two. Choice B is mentioned as a criticism of the dialectical viewpoint, but it is not the primary focus of the passage. Marx's view of capitalism (choice C) is mentioned merely in passing and is not the main point of the passage. Choice D is correct because the author describes a viewpoint, details an objection to it, and then discusses how that objection may be overcome.

47. **The correct answer is D.** This question requires you to find the main idea. The passage discusses living fossils, a term biologists use to designate a species that has changed little since its inception. It then provides details on four different living fossils. Choice D is the best description of the passage. The passage doesn't primarily explain how these species remain unchanged as choice A states. Nor does it detail a dilemma (choice B) or focus mainly on the coelacanth (choice C).

48. **The correct answer is B.** In order to answer this question, you must choose an accurate paraphrase of the information in the passage. The first paragraph states

that living fossils are not primitive. Rather they are so well adapted to their environment that there is little need for change. Thinking that evolution necessarily represents advancement is indeed a misunderstanding, as choice B indicates. Choice A is not what the passage states as there is no comparison to other species. Choice C may be true, but it doesn't answer the question. Choice D is not stated in the passage.

49. **The correct answer is C.** This question asks you to solve a problem. Here, you need to use information from the passage to put the time periods in the correct order. The discussion of the horseshoe crab indicates that the Jurassic period is the most recent, some 200 million years ago. The Permian period, at which time the lungfish ceased experiencing major evolutionary changes, was about 250 million years ago. And the Silurian period, from which the coelacanth emerged, was more than 400 million years ago. That makes choice C the best answer.

50. **The correct answer is A.** You need to analyze an argument in order to answer this question. In the context of the passage, in which the majority of the information explains that living fossils have changed very little, why would the author include a part about rapid evolutionary change? The answer is to show that a living fossil does change and evolve; however, the changes are minor or cease at some point. Choice A is the best answer.

51. **The correct answer is A.** This question requires you to draw conclusions. The author does not state choice A explicitly, but does say that the discovery was aided by an "astounding coincidence." The passage indicates that biologists find the lungfish interesting, but that does not necessarily imply the author believes the same as choice B says. Choice C is not a valid conclusion based on the passage. The author indicates that the discovery of the coelacanth was a major surprise, but that doesn't mean that biologists were wrong to believe it was extinct. There is no evidence to support choice D.

52. **The correct answer is D.** This question asks you to compare and contrast information found in the passage. We know from the second paragraph that the horseshoe crab is the most recent living fossil at 200 million years old. The other three all date from around 400 million years ago. The final paragraph says that at that time, land-dwelling plants were just beginning to evolve. Thus, choice D is the best answer because the land-dwelling plants had been evolving for about 200 million years by the time the horseshoe crab appeared on the scene. Choices A and B indicate aspects the crab shares with some of the other living fossils. There is no evidence of choice C.

53. **The correct answer is A.** This question tests your ability to analyze an argument. The last paragraph continually emphasizes how the discovery of the coelacanth was an amazing event. The author uses words like *singular, astounding*, and *surprising*. This corresponds to choice A. There is no evidence for choice B or D, and

the paragraph does not make it clear that it is the public who reacted with the allegations as choice C indicates.

54. **The correct answer is C.** To answer this question, you must apply new evidence. According to the passage, a living fossil is one that has changed very little over the eons. In order to argue that the coelacanth is not a living fossil, a biologist would need to find evidence of significant change. Showing that the coelacanth actually comes from a different line, as choice C does, would do so. The age of the species is not the issue, as choices A and D indicate. And finding different species, as in choice B, would not affect the status of the coelacanth as a living fossil.

55. **The correct answer is C.** This question asks you to choose an accurate paraphrase. The first paragraph explains what puzzles political scientists so look back at it and try to put the information into your own words. The author states that common-sense explanations of what motivates voters are generally correct, so choice A is wrong. The problem lies instead with why people expend the time and energy to vote when they could reap the benefits without voting and when it is unlikely that their votes will have an impact as choice C, the best answer, states.

56. **The correct answer is B.** You must draw a conclusion to answer this question. The thought expressed in the final sentence of the first paragraph is most similar to what a free rider would believe; namely, a free rider wants to enjoy the benefits of something without incurring the costs. So the best answer is choice B.

57. **The correct answer is A.** To answer this question, you must make a generalization. The passage states that those individuals with more resources are more likely to vote. Of the answers, choice A is best. Lawyers have high levels of education and tend to make a fair amount of money. Choice D might be tempting, but it isn't clear what the education level of the homemaker is, making choice A better. Also, the passage states that Switzerland and the United States have low voter turnout numbers, which eliminates choices B and C.

58. **The correct answer is C.** This question requires you to analyze an argument. Looking back at the passage, the author identifies three main explanatory factors: resources, mobilization, and instrumental motivation. Assertion I is incorrect because the passage does not state a person needs "large amounts" of free time; a person simply needs enough time to vote. Assertion II would correspond to a mobilization factor, while assertion III indicates a level of instrumental motivation. Thus, choice C is the best answer.

59. **The correct answer is A.** This is a fairly straightforward question that asks about supporting details. In the final paragraph, the author states that the baseline model "achieves some success . . . but is useless" when trying to compare voting behavior among citizens of different countries. Of the answers, choice A best states this. Choice B is wrong because it is too general. As the passage states, the model only works in certain cases. There is no evidence to support choice C or D.

60. **The correct answer is D.** A question that asks what the passage implies is asking you to draw conclusions. The correct answer will not be directly stated, so you'll have to look at what inference you can draw from the given information. Choice A cannot be inferred. The passage states that the theory of baseline political participation holds that resources are the key factor, but this theory is shown to be deficient. Choice B is also incorrect. The author states that resources have received the "most scholarly attention," but that doesn't mean the other two factors have been ignored. There is no support for choice C either, since the author only addresses one theory that has been found lacking. That leaves choice D, the correct answer. The author states that resources have received the most attention, so that implies mobilization has received less attention.

EVALUATION CHART

Use this Evaluation Chart to analyze your results on the science sections (Sections 1, 2, and 3) of Practice Test 2. Check the Answers and Explanations section to see which answers you got correct and which ones you missed. For each question that you missed, find the question number in the left column of the chart below. Look in the right column to see the chapter in a companion volume in the **McGraw-Hill Education MCAT Test Preparation series** that covers the content area for that question. If you missed questions in a specific content area, you need to pay particular attention to that area as you study for the MCAT.

Item Number	Content Area
Biological and Biochemical Foundations of Living Systems	
	Chapter in *McGraw-Hill Education: MCAT Biological and Biochemical Foundations of Living Systems*
1.	Chapter 9: Structure and Integrative Functions of the Main Organ Systems
2.	Chapter 9: Structure and Integrative Functions of the Main Organ Systems
3.	Chapter 4: Principles of Bioenergetics and Fuel Molecule Metabolism
4.	Chapter 5: Assemblies of Molecules, Cells, and Groups of Cells Within Multicellular Organisms
5.	Chapter 9: Structure and Integrative Functions of the Main Organ Systems
6.	Chapter 5: Assemblies of Molecules, Cells, and Groups of Cells Within Multicellular Organisms
7.	Chapter 3: Transmission of Heritable Information from Generation to Generation and the Processes That Increase Genetic Diversity
8.	Chapter 7: Processes of Cell Division, Differentiation, and Specialization
9.	Chapter 7: Processes of Cell Division, Differentiation, and Specialization
10.	Chapter 3: Transmission of Heritable Information from Generation to Generation and the Processes That Increase Genetic Diversity
11.	Chapter 3: Transmission of Heritable Information from Generation to Generation and the Processes That Increase Genetic Diversity
12.	Chapter 9: Structure and Integrative Functions of the Main Organ Systems
13.	Chapter 9: Structure and Integrative Functions of the Main Organ Systems
14.	Chapter 8: Structure and Function of the Nervous and Endocrine Systems and Ways in Which These Systems Coordinate the Organ Systems
15.	Chapter 8: Structure and Function of the Nervous and Endocrine Systems and Ways in Which These Systems Coordinate the Organ Systems
16.	Chapter 8: Structure and Function of the Nervous and Endocrine Systems and Ways in Which These Systems Coordinate the Organ Systems
17.	Chapter 9: Structure and Integrative Functions of the Main Organ Systems
18.	Chapter 9: Structure and Integrative Functions of the Main Organ Systems
19.	Chapter 7: Processes of Cell Division, Differentiation, and Specialization
20.	Chapter 7: Processes of Cell Division, Differentiation, and Specialization
21.	Chapter 7: Processes of Cell Division, Differentiation, and Specialization

(Continued)

Item Number	Content Area
22.	Chapter 9: Structure and Integrative Functions of the Main Organ Systems
23.	Chapter 7: Processes of Cell Division, Differentiation, and Specialization
24.	Chapter 9: Structure and Integrative Functions of the Main Organ Systems
25.	Chapter 9: Structure and Integrative Functions of the Main Organ Systems
26.	Chapter 2: Transmission of Genetic Information from the Gene to the Protein
27.	Chapter 9: Structure and Integrative Functions of the Main Organ Systems
28.	Chapter 1: Structure and Function of Proteins and Their Constituent Amino Acids
29.	Chapter 9: Structure and Integrative Functions of the Main Organ Systems
30.	Chapter 9: Structure and Integrative Functions of the Main Organ Systems
31.	Chapter 9: Structure and Integrative Functions of the Main Organ Systems
32.	Chapter 9: Structure and Integrative Functions of the Main Organ Systems
33.	Chapter 2: Transmission of Genetic Information from the Gene to the Protein
34.	Chapter 9: Structure and Integrative Functions of the Main Organ Systems
35.	Chapter 6: Structure, Growth, Physiology, and Genetics of Prokaryotes and Viruses
36.	Chapter 9: Structure and Integrative Functions of the Main Organ Systems
37.	Chapter 8: Structure and Function of the Nervous and Endocrine Systems and Ways in Which These Systems Coordinate the Organ Systems
38.	Chapter 6: Structure, Growth, Physiology, and Genetics of Prokaryotes and Viruses
39.	Chapter 2: Transmission of Genetic Information from the Gene to the Protein
40.	Chapter 6: Structure, Growth, Physiology, and Genetics of Prokaryotes and Viruses
41.	Chapter 1: Structure and Function of Proteins and Their Constituent Amino Acids
42.	Chapter 6: Structure, Growth, Physiology, and Genetics of Prokaryotes and Viruses
43.	Chapter 5: Assemblies of Molecules, Cells, and Groups of Cells Within Multicellular Organisms
44.	Chapter 5: Assemblies of Molecules, Cells, and Groups of Cells Within Multicellular Organisms
45.	Chapter 5: Assemblies of Molecules, Cells, and Groups of Cells Within Multicellular Organisms
46.	Chapter 4: Principles of Bioenergetics and Fuel Molecule Metabolism
47.	Chapter 5: Assemblies of Molecules, Cells, and Groups of Cells Within Multicellular Organisms
48.	Chapter 5: Assemblies of Molecules, Cells, and Groups of Cells Within Multicellular Organisms
49.	Chapter 2: Transmission of Genetic Information from the Gene to the Protein
50.	Chapter 2: Transmission of Genetic Information from the Gene to the Protein
51.	Chapter 2: Transmission of Genetic Information from the Gene to the Protein
52.	Chapter 5: Assemblies of Molecules, Cells, and Groups of Cells Within Multicellular Organisms
53.	Chapter 9: Structure and Integrative Functions of the Main Organ Systems
54.	Chapter 2: Transmission of Genetic Information from the Gene to the Protein
55.	Chapter 9: Structure and Integrative Functions of the Main Organ Systems
56.	Chapter 9: Structure and Integrative Functions of the Main Organ Systems
57.	Chapter 9: Structure and Integrative Functions of the Main Organ Systems
58.	Chapter 9: Structure and Integrative Functions of the Main Organ Systems
59.	Chapter 9: Structure and Integrative Functions of the Main Organ Systems
60.	Chapter 5: Assemblies of Molecules, Cells, and Groups of Cells Within Multicellular Organisms

Item Number	Content Area
61.	Chapter 1: Structure and Function of Proteins and Their Constituent Amino Acids
62.	Chapter 5: Assemblies of Molecules, Cells, and Groups of Cells Within Multicellular Organisms
63.	Chapter 4: Principles of Bioenergetics and Fuel Molecule Metabolism
64.	Chapter 3: Transmission of Heritable Information from Generation to Generation and the Processes That Increase Genetic Diversity
65.	Chapter 8: Structure and Function of the Nervous and Endocrine Systems and Ways in Which These Systems Coordinate the Organ Systems

Chemical and Physical Foundations of Biological Systems

Chapter in *McGraw-Hill Education: MCAT Chemical and Physical Foundations of Biological Systems*

1.	Chapter 10: Translational Motion, Forces, Work, Energy, and Equilibrium in Living Systems
2.	Chapter 12: Electrochemistry and Electrical Circuits and Their Elements
3.	Chapter 18: Structure, Function, and Reactivity of Biologically-Relevant Molecules
4.	Chapter 18: Structure, Function, and Reactivity of Biologically-Relevant Molecules
5.	Chapter 18: Structure, Function, and Reactivity of Biologically-Relevant Molecules
6.	Chapter 18: Structure, Function, and Reactivity of Biologically-Relevant Molecules
7.	Chapter 18: Structure, Function, and Reactivity of Biologically-Relevant Molecules
8.	Chapter 10: Translational Motion, Forces, Work, Energy, and Equilibrium in Living Systems
9.	Chapter 10: Translational Motion, Forces, Work, Energy, and Equilibrium in Living Systems
10.	Chapter 10: Translational Motion, Forces, Work, Energy, and Equilibrium in Living Systems
11.	Chapter 10: Translational Motion, Forces, Work, Energy, and Equilibrium in Living Systems
12.	Chapter 10: Translational Motion, Forces, Work, Energy, and Equilibrium in Living Systems
13.	Chapter 10: Translational Motion, Forces, Work, Energy, and Equilibrium in Living Systems
14.	Chapter 10: Translational Motion, Forces, Work, Energy, and Equilibrium in Living Systems
15.	Chapter 17: Separation and Purification Methods Chapter 18: Structure, Function, and Reactivity of Biologically-Relevant Molecules
16.	Chapter 17: Separation and Purification Methods Chapter 18: Structure, Function, and Reactivity of Biologically-Relevant Molecules
17.	Chapter 17: Separation and Purification Methods Chapter 18: Structure, Function, and Reactivity of Biologically-Relevant Molecules
18.	Chapter 17: Separation and Purification Methods Chapter 18: Structure, Function, and Reactivity of Biologically-Relevant Molecules

(Continued)

Item Number	Content Area
19.	Chapter 17: Separation and Purification Methods Chapter 18: Structure, Function, and Reactivity of Biologically-Relevant Molecules
20.	Chapter 10: Translational Motion, Forces, Work, Energy, and Equilibrium in Living Systems
21.	Chapter 10: Translational Motion, Forces, Work, Energy, and Equilibrium in Living Systems
22.	Chapter 10: Translational Motion, Forces, Work, Energy, and Equilibrium in Living Systems
23.	Chapter 10: Translational Motion, Forces, Work, Energy, and Equilibrium in Living Systems
24.	Chapter 10: Translational Motion, Forces, Work, Energy, and Equilibrium in Living Systems
25.	Chapter 10: Translational Motion, Forces, Work, Energy, and Equilibrium in Living Systems
26.	Chapter 18: Structure, Function, and Reactivity of Biologically-Relevant Molecules
27.	Chapter 17: Separation and Purification Methods Chapter 18: Structure, Function, and Reactivity of Biologically-Relevant Molecules
28.	Chapter 17: Separation and Purification Methods Chapter 18: Structure, Function, and Reactivity of Biologically-Relevant Molecules
29.	Chapter 17: Separation and Purification Methods Chapter 18: Structure, Function, and Reactivity of Biologically-Relevant Molecules
30.	Chapter 17: Separation and Purification Methods Chapter 18: Structure, Function, and Reactivity of Biologically-Relevant Molecules
31.	Chapter 18: Structure, Function, and Reactivity of Biologically-Relevant Molecules
32.	Chapter 12: Electrochemistry and Electrical Circuits and Their Elements
33.	Chapter 13: How Light and Sound Interact with Matter
34.	Chapter 14: Atoms, Nuclear Decay, Electronic Structure, and Atomic Chemical Behavior
35.	Chapter 15: Unique Nature of Water and Its Solutions Chapter 16: Nature of Molecules and Intermolecular Interactions Chapter 19: Principles of Chemical Thermodynamics and Kinetics
36.	Chapter 15: Unique Nature of Water and Its Solutions Chapter 16: Nature of Molecules and Intermolecular Interactions
37.	Chapter 15: Unique Nature of Water and Its Solutions Chapter 16: Nature of Molecules and Intermolecular Interactions
38.	Chapter 16: Nature of Molecules and Intermolecular Interactions
39.	Chapter 16: Nature of Molecules and Intermolecular Interactions
40.	Chapter 11: Importance of Fluids for the Circulation of Blood, Gas Movement, and Gas Exchange
41.	Chapter 11: Importance of Fluids for the Circulation of Blood, Gas Movement, and Gas Exchange
42.	Chapter 11: Importance of Fluids for the Circulation of Blood, Gas Movement, and Gas Exchange
43.	Chapter 11: Importance of Fluids for the Circulation of Blood, Gas Movement, and Gas Exchange

Item Number	Content Area
44.	Chapter 11: Importance of Fluids for the Circulation of Blood, Gas Movement, and Gas Exchange
45.	Chapter 18: Structure, Function, and Reactivity of Biologically-Relevant Molecules
46.	Chapter 18: Structure, Function, and Reactivity of Biologically-Relevant Molecules
47.	Chapter 18: Structure, Function, and Reactivity of Biologically-Relevant Molecules
48.	Chapter 18: Structure, Function, and Reactivity of Biologically-Relevant Molecules
49.	Chapter 18: Structure, Function, and Reactivity of Biologically-Relevant Molecules
50.	Chapter 13: How Light and Sound Interact with Matter
51.	Chapter 13: How Light and Sound Interact with Matter
52.	Chapter 13: How Light and Sound Interact with Matter
53.	Chapter 13: How Light and Sound Interact with Matter
54.	Chapter 13: How Light and Sound Interact with Matter
55.	Chapter 19: Principles of Chemical Thermodynamics and Kinetics
56.	Chapter 19: Principles of Chemical Thermodynamics and Kinetics
57.	Chapter 19: Principles of Chemical Thermodynamics and Kinetics
58.	Chapter 19: Principles of Chemical Thermodynamics and Kinetics
59.	Chapter 19: Principles of Chemical Thermodynamics and Kinetics
60.	Chapter 19: Principles of Chemical Thermodynamics and Kinetics
61.	Chapter 18: Structure, Function, and Reactivity of Biologically-Relevant Molecules
62.	Chapter 18: Structure, Function, and Reactivity of Biologically-Relevant Molecules
63.	Chapter 18: Structure, Function, and Reactivity of Biologically-Relevant Molecules
64.	Chapter 18: Structure, Function, and Reactivity of Biologically-Relevant Molecules
65.	Chapter 18: Structure, Function, and Reactivity of Biologically-Relevant Molecules

Psychological, Social, and Biological Foundations of Behavior

	Chapter in *McGraw-Hill Education: MCAT Behavioral and Social Sciences & Critical Analysis*
1.	Chapter 9: Romantic Attraction
2.	Chapter 2: Language: Different Brain Areas Control Language and Speech
3.	Chapter 12: Theories of Stratification
4.	Chapter 4: Attitudes
5.	Chapter 12: Theories of Stratification
6.	Chapter 1: Vision: Visual Processing
7.	Chapter 1: Vision: Visual Processing
8.	Chapter 1: Vision: Visual Processing
9.	Chapter 1: Vision: Visual Processing
10.	Chapter 1: Vision: Visual Processing
11.	Chapter 9: Romantic Attraction
12.	Chapter 9: Romantic Attraction
13.	Chapter 9: Romantic Attraction

Item Number	Content Area
14.	Chapter 9: Romantic Attraction
15.	Chapter 9: Romantic Attraction
16.	Chapter 2: Memory: Encoding
17.	Chapter 2: Memory
18.	Chapter 2: Memory
19.	Chapter 2: Memory: Information Processing in the Cerebral Cortex
20.	Chapter 2: Memory: Information Processing in the Cerebral Cortex
21.	Chapter 2: Memory
22.	Chapter 2: Memory
23.	Chapter 2: Memory
24.	Chapter 2: Memory
25.	Chapter 2: Memory
26.	Chapter 4: Personality
27.	Chapter 4: Personality
28.	Chapter 4: Personality
29.	Chapter 4: Personality
30.	Chapter 4: Personality
31.	Chapter 12: Theories of Stratification/Poverty
32.	Chapter 12: Theories of Stratification/Poverty
33.	Chapter 12: Theories of Stratification/Poverty
34.	Chapter 12: Theories of Stratification/Poverty
35.	Chapter 12: Theories of Stratification/Poverty
36.	Chapter 4: Psychological Disorders
37.	Chapter 4: Psychological Disorders
38.	Chapter 4: Psychological Disorders
39.	Chapter 4: Psychological Disorders
40.	Chapter 4: Psychological Disorders
41.	Chapter 4: Sleep
42.	Chapter 4: Sleep
43.	Chapter 4: Sleep
44.	Chapter 4: Sleep
45.	Chapter 4: Sleep
46.	Chapter 5: How Groups Affect Individuals
47.	Chapter 5: How Groups Affect Individuals
48.	Chapter 5: How Groups Affect Individuals
49.	Chapter 5: How Groups Affect Individuals
50.	Chapter 5: How Groups Affect Individuals
51.	Chapter 4: Attitudes/Socialization
52.	Chapter 4: Attitudes/Socialization
53.	Chapter 4: Attitudes/Socialization
54.	Chapter 4: Attitudes/Socialization
55.	Chapter 4: Attitudes/Socialization
56.	Chapter 3: Stress
57.	Chapter 3: Stress
58.	Chapter 3: Stress
59.	Chapter 3: Stress
60.	Chapter 3: Stress
61.	Chapter 10: Social Structure/Social Institutions
62.	Chapter 10: Social Structure/Social Institutions
63.	Chapter 10: Social Structure/Social Institutions
64.	Chapter 10: Social Structure/Social Institutions
65.	Chapter 10: Social Structure/Social Institutions